BEFORE, DURING, & AFTER MENOPAUSE

YOUR RESOURCE GUIDE TO *CRUISING* THROUGH MENOPAUSE
WITH GRACE, GRATITUDE, CONFIDENCE, AND EASE

Gwen Harris
and the Menopause Support Group
Council of Experts

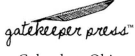

gatekeeper press™

Columbus, Ohio

Before, During, and After Menopause: Your Resource Guide to *Cruising* Through Menopause with Grace, Gratitude, Confidence, and Ease

Published by Gatekeeper Press
2167 Stringtown Rd, Suite 109
Columbus, OH 43123-2989
www.GatekeeperPress.com

ISBN (paperback): 9781662906053

DEDICATION

To Women Worldwide on the Journey of Menopause!
May we experience it with grace, gratitude, confidence and ease!

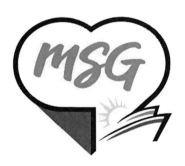

TABLE OF CONTENTS

If you're a woman going through menopause, or you're the mother, daughter, husband or friend of someone going through menopause, you need this book! The information is essential and it's all delivered with love and humor throughout. Gwen Harris has gathered a group of incredible women, each a leading expert in their own field, and each with a shared story about their personal experience with Menopause. They share advice on life coaching, fitness and nutrition, even money management, astrology and, most importantly, happiness. They explain new methods and products to help you manage this changing and important chapter of your life. Gwen calls it MSG, the Menopause Support Group. Remember, you're not alone! I highly recommend this book.

Casey Maxwell Clair
Casey Maxwell Clair enjoyed a career as a successful comedy writer and television producer on many popular sit-coms. She is also the author of the acclaimed memoir
AN ONLY CHILD AND HER SISTER: A true Hollywood story.
caseymaxwellclair.com

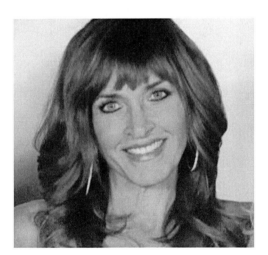

Gwen Harris

INTRODUCTION

Seven years ago, it hit me like a monsoon; horrible soaking sweats, day and night. I had to keep extra clothes in my car in case I broke out into that dreaded, sticky sweat during the day. My sleep at night was interrupted because I would wake up drenched and needed to change the sheets. I drank a gallon of water every day, but the constant lack of hydration left my skin feeling like the parched sand in a desert. No amount of lotion soothed my itchy, cracked skin. The most painful affliction I suffered from was the pain in my eyes. When I opened them in the morning, I felt like I was being stabbed in the pupil. This loss of hydration, hormone changes and reduced tear production caused my eyelids to literally glue themselves to my eyeball, so when I opened them in the morning, the film on my eye would tear. On top of being in the drudges of menopause, I was now diagnosed with corneal erosions.

It was really starting to hit me hard. Here I was, only fifty-four years young, and I felt alone, suffering in this invisible bubble called menopause. Who did I talk to? Was I the only one who felt this way? Will I be this exhausted the rest of my life since I never get a good night's sleep? Am I going to forever feel stinky from these persistent soaking sweats? I eat organically and exercise, yet I feel like I'm caught in perpetual vortex called the menopausal plague.

I didn't know where to turn. Who do I dare talk to about this? NO ONE talks about menopause. Calgon...TAKE ME AWAY!!!!

That wasn't likely to happen. I tried many a cool soothing bath but like hot fudge on an ice cream sundae, those dreaded soaking sweats immediately poured over me.

I sought care from an ophthalmologist for my eyes and turned to a female naturopath for everything else. They were helpful, BUT I still felt alone and curious if others were suffering my predicament, Out of total despair, I decided to start a Facebook group called The Menopause Support Group to see if anyone else on the planet was struggling too. To my surprise, the group grew to 11,000 members in five years. Clearly, I wasn't alone in my struggles. Although women suffer a myriad of pain points in menopause, I felt comforted knowing I wasn't alone. To me, this brought comfort.

On a sunny Seattle day in January 2018…you're right, that doesn't happen often…I was out hiking with a friend and received a message via FB messenger. The message said, "Gwen, I am a producer for the Good Morning America Show. We are going to be doing a weeklong series on menopause. These days, we seek content on social media and saw you had a large menopause support group of 11,000 members. We would like to speak with you and feature you on the show."

Yeah, right, I thought. It could just as easily be a scam.

I showed the message to my friend and my husband, who both said, "Be careful, but go for it. They have the facts straight and this could be a thing." I responded by asking them to give me their phone number and a good time to call them.

Two days later, I called at the specified time and they answered with, "ABC News, how can we help you?" I asked to be transferred to the producer who messaged me and was promptly connected. She answered the phone and, my goodness, this was the real deal.

About a week later, ABC news sent their film crew to my home. They spent the better part of a day with me, and we were ultimately featured on Good Morning America.

Fast forward to December 2019, The Menopause Support group has grown to 60,000 members in 120 countries and continues to grow by hundreds every day.

During the summer of 2018, as the group exploded, women from all over the world, asked me to plan conventions so we could meet. The thought of planning such an event terrified me and I wondered, "How will this serve women globally? I doubt women from Singapore, India, Bali or South Africa will come to a convention in America."

September 2018 introduced a season of debilitating fear. I rolled over in bed one night and felt the worst pain I've ever felt. It shot through my body, resonating from my back like a strike of lightning. I went to an orthopedic surgeon and after an MRI was told I need multiple fusions, multiple laminectomies and bone grafts. Just what I needed to hear. Three subsequent professional opinions confirmed the diagnosis and on 12/13/19 I had invasive back surgery. By this time, I lost had complete use of my left leg. Seriously, I am a hiker. I am active. I "kind of" conquered the menopause symptoms and NOW THIS!!!

Halfway during surgery, my surgeon told my husband that he didn't expect me to regain use of my left leg. My nerves had been so compressed that they were "as flat as ribbons" and he didn't expect them to recover.

Despite this bleak prognosis, surgery in itself was a success and the magnificent metal structure in my back, known as a "cage" was securely in place, holding everything together. I was in the hospital a week then sent home to recover, without the use of my left leg.

Recovery was debilitating but rich. I had been forced to "Be still and know that He is God." This kind of stillness isn't what I bargained for.

After all, I had a global network of women who were counting on me to plan a convention and build a supportive menopause community. I had plans and they included me being healthy and whole. All I did was roll over in bed and my entire back snapped. God, what are you doing with me? He forced me to be still so I could reflect on what He had in mind.

During those arduous months of recovery, I thought, *why not plan menopause support group cruises? Ships cruise all over the world and that way we could bless all our members.* Harris Holiday Cruises, to host the special event cruises for my menopause support group was born in May 2019, during recovery from my back surgery.

I announced out first cruise in the group, which was a 7-day cruise in September 2019 to Alaska, embarking from Seattle. I had NO IDEA what to expect. I had booked the space for our menopause sisterhood cruise, but who was going to support me? Who would help me with the events? My dearest friend, Anjl Rodee, an icon and true female force, rallied beside me and encouraged me to keep on keeping on.

She vowed to support me and said, "The right people will show up." She knew what she was talking about, and before I knew it, Sandy Hartwell of Hartwell Fitness and Dr. Maria Maricich, of The Wellness Clinic, both members of my menopause group, reached out to join my vision, that being to educate and inspire women to embrace life's transitional seasons with grace, gratitude, confidence and ease.

The first cruise exceeded all expectations. We had women from around the world join us. Our on-board private events included presentations by our experts, an evening of paint therapy, entertainment and comedy, a night of inspiration and of course, lifelong friendships that were made. I knew this was another beginning of something huge and that moving forward, indeed, I needed to plan cruises all over the world so we could include as many women as possible. I also knew our team of experts needed to grow and that's exactly what happened. As pictures from the cruise and personal stories were shared, members of the group who are experts in their subsequent professions reached out to me. They aligned with my vision and wanted to step up and serve. I couldn't have written a better business plan. Not one expert who is on our council competes with another. They all complimented one another and each offer solutions for a myriad of menopausal pain points.

When Dr. Anita M. Jackson joined our council of experts, I shared my vision of starting a scholarship fund that would bless women who couldn't afford the entire cost of a cruise. As an author and publisher, she immediately suggested that a book be written, and the proceeds used to establish that fund. This is that book.

Our experts each authored a chapter in the book. They briefly share their menopausal journey and write about their expertise. This tremendous resource will offer you solutions for your menopausal symptoms. Each expert has the global capability to coach and offer their services.

My desire is to bless each of you with the best care possible. Our experts will do just that.

Gwen Harris
Founder and CEO
Harris Holiday Cruises

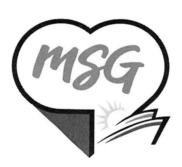

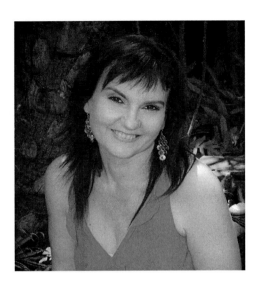

Susanne McAllister

When an intriguing message comes to you from down under, you give it immediate consideration. That's precisely what I did. I was compelled by Susanne's credentials and needed to know her story.

Susanne possesses an inner force that has transformed her personal misfortunes into a vehicle for empowerment.

After the unforeseen premature death of her husband that left her as a single mother in midlife, she knew she had to "stay the course" for her daughters.

An accredited psychotherapist, Susanne chose to focus on women's issues. "I knew this was not the time for me to give up, but instead, turn this personal tribulation into victory. Living in numerous international countries, I've seen how women all over the world suffer, and now here I was. It was now or never."

Susanne is a consummate author, an inquisitive student, a tenderhearted life-coach and a devoted mother. To know her is to know a friend for life.

FEELING LOST? TIPS TO CRACKING THE MENOPAUSE CODE

By Susanne McAllister

I F YOU ARE A little bit like me, you might have spent a lot of your time over the last twenty or so years taking care of others. Others, like your children, your husband / partner and / or your career. After the death of my husband seven years ago, I was the sole provider and sole parent for my teenage girls, then aged twelve and sixteen. Having had a less than desirable childhood myself, I was a woman on a mission. I wanted the least damage and pain as possible for my daughters Caroline and Gabriella, no matter what!

I poured my heart and soul into learning all the things my husband had done for us all these years. I had always been the spiritual warm and caring mum that loved to study anything that involved self-development, spirituality and health. My husband was the businessman who did the taxes and paid the bills. He truly was my soulmate and the two years of his cancer battle proved to be a very hard time for our little close-knit family. We had chosen to live at the other end of the world in Australia, with no family. All we had was each other plus a handful of close friends that would forever be grateful for.

I thought I was doing okay, then my oldest daughter moved out to study and that really did hit me hard. But when my youngest daughter turned eighteen, I hit a new low. I experienced total burnout, menopause, and then empty nest syndrome knocked me off my feet! I knew something was seriously wrong when one day I was asked for my address and I couldn't even remember my house number!

I thought I was experiencing the early onset of Alzheimer's or that there was something seriously wrong with my brain. I felt so low in energy. I felt like crying a lot of the time and in the next minute I would be in a rage! I never slept and I always worried.

What Helped?

I was already a practicing nutritional therapist, helping women to optimize their health, lose weight the healthy and holistic way, and find their passion in life. I was combining positive psychology and mindfulness with supplements, real food and Inner Connection Process (ICT for short. It is a process I had developed when I worked as clinical hypnotherapist). It was time to take my own medicine and to do some serious work on myself. I had to use all the tools that I had learned during the previous twenty-five years and pull them together to heal myself.

Not only did I finally lose the extra twenty-five pounds I had been carrying around for years, but I also found a new way of living. I had re-invented myself and my life and had learned how to take care of myself. I have walked this road, just a few steps in front of you and I would love to be your guide, if you are going through something similar. This is how my book **With Sex, NO drugs and Rock'n Roll through Menopause and Beyond** was born. This book is a self-help guide focusing on life during and after menopause, including natural remedies, a guide to Tantra, and it even includes chapters for men who support menopausal women.

I really don't want for you the fear, dread, and uncertainty that surrounds your menopause and it is definitely not true that your best years are behind you.

My book guides the reader through menopause naturally and offers a range of advice for physical, mental, spiritual, and even sexual health.

Here are few examples of what you will find in the book, in addition to the many simple strategies and cutting-edge information:

▶ Tests you really need to know about and questions to ask your Doctor

- ► To HRT or not to HRT?
- ► Common Challenges and what really helps
- ► Which Supplements and Homeopathic remedies to take and why
- ► The emotional impact of Menopause and what to do
- ► How you can keep your symptoms at bay with Hypnosis – breathe – and mind-control
- ► A Low Tox Life for your Body and Home
- ► Essential Oils for menopause
- ► Addressing brain fog naturally
- ► A whole chapter for the BOYS – how your man can help
- ► How to finally make peace with your body
- ► Let's talk about sex, baby! Tantra is not a dirty word!

But just writing a book was not enough. I really wanted to create a one-stop-shop for women who are looking to go through menopause as naturally as possible. This is how my naturally wise women forty plus lifestyle membership was born. I wanted to reach as many women as possible. There is nothing that brings me more joy than to witness the transformation of a woman who feels alone and past it to a woman who is glowing with confidence and new love for her body and life. And yes, before you ask, this is possible for you too! I know, because I did it and so can you! You've got this! But stop trying to figure this out on your own! Let me and other women in our tribe be your guides.

The naturally wise women lifestyle membership has it all figured out for you! Every month we have a different theme that will be super helpful as you are going through this season in your life. You get a tailored meal plan (mainstream/vegan/weight loss) with a shopping list to help take the frustration and guesswork out of what to cook to support your body.

Every month we tackle a different part of menopause, sometimes it's all about curing the pesky symptoms like hot flashes or not sleeping naturally and it is always with a complete mind, body and spirited approach. Often, we know what we should eat or do, but our emotions and cravings get the better of us. In the tribe, I teach you how to not to eat your emotions and how to outsmart your cravings.

Every month there is mindfulness and movement video training that will help you move your body YOUR body's way and develop a calm and peaceful mind no matter what.

We are doing meetups, organising events and our cruises all over the world for you to connect to your tribe face to face. I have also launched the "naturally wise women 40+" podcast, where you can listen to interviews with experts from around the world full of fun advice on how to get through menopause and the midlife transition naturally and holistically.

This is your time now!
It is time to re-discover YOU!
Time to develop a new Sense of Self!

Questions to Ask Yourself.

These are just some of the questions that we figure out together in the tribe. Why not grab a pen and paper and write down what comes to your heart and mind?

- ► Who are you now?
- ► How have your relationships changed?
- ► Maybe you are single for the first time in many years or you are looking at your spouse, wondering what has happened to your relationship and your love life?
- ► How are you feeling about your changing body?
- ► What things do you say to yourself in your mind?
- ► Who makes up your tribe? Do they inspire you?
- ► What are the new roles that you would like to play in this season of your life beyond being a mum and beyond being a wife or a woman that is solo or single?

And there are also your parents to consider, if you are lucky enough that they are still around. On one side, you may have children that still need / or not need you, and then on the other side you may have your parents going through their own ageing struggles, needing your help also.

The only thing we really have control over, is who we want to be through all of this. How do we want to respond to all of life's challenges? How can you be a naturally wise women through all of this, content and happy within herself?

Please also, let me congratulate you. You are a woman looking for change, a woman who is limitless, a woman who wants to live her best life or you wouldn't be reading this. Not everyone sets out to find themselves during this time in their life! So, thank you for being here with me.

Be kind and gentle with yourself and learn how to be YOUR BEST FRIEND. Turn your attention and intention inward and get to know yourself as a *wise woman*.

How Can You Do This?

Well, of course I would recommend to you to join my naturally wise women forty plus lifestyle membership! For a small monthly subscription, you get all the tools to get through menopause naturally and holistically in JOY and community. You never have to wonder what to cook, how to deal with your emotions and cravings, you learn how to combat the most common symptoms naturally, you learn how to move your body – your body's way and how to calm your mind. You learn how to re-invent your life and live your passion and feel happy, healthy and strong again.

Here are just a few helpful techniques we use in the tribe to get you started:

Learn how to use mindfulness to purposefully focus on our present world, including; awareness of our feelings, thoughts, bodily sensations, and our environment with a non-judgmental lens. What a relief it is, when the super critical inner critique has said goodbye to us.

When you practice mindfulness, you accept what you are feeling and experiencing and pay attention to your emotions without judgment. There is no right or wrong when it comes to your feelings, and you simply learn to feel them in the present moment.

Mindfulness is vital to your emotional health in many ways. First, it teaches you to be more self-aware, which allows you to understand better the emotions you are feeling.

Second, it provides you with insight into how your emotions are affecting your physical and mental state. Mindfulness keeps you grounded in the present, which prevents unproductive worry about the future or rehashing of past events.

Mindfulness is a wonderful way to cope with stress, as well. It allows you to process what you are feeling so that you can deal with these emotions and move forward rather than stewing in your ongoing concerns and fears.

We have a new mindfulness exercise for you in the tribe.

Here is the link to a free taster for you: https://www.susannemcallister.com/mindfulness

The tribe is based on the principal of positive psychology, which focuses on helping you understand what it is that makes you happy while teaching you strategies to attain that happiness in your life. The focus of positive psychology is teaching you how to cultivate positive emotions, including contentment, joy, and hope while also developing positive traits. These traits include self-knowledge, compassion, creativity, curiosity, resilience, and courage.

Positive psychology is not positive thinking but instead a more holistic approach to thinking and reasoning that allows you to learn from your emotions instead of just trying to be optimistic all the time.

Let's focus in on a couple of emotions that many women experience during menopause and let me give you a few practical tips.

Many women also experience more anxiety and mood swings during menopause.

Here are my top tips to get you started to manage your emotions during menopause:

- ▶ Make sure you eat a diet with healthy, nutritiously dense foods in it. Avoid processed foods and foods containing things like sugar, salt, and high fructose corn syrup. I have a free 7-day meal plan here for you www.susannemcallister.com so you can try it straight away.

▶ Eat smaller portions. If you get food cravings, try eating a small snack instead of loading up on unhealthy foods.

▶ Take in at least five portions of vegetables per day and at least two servings of fruit per day. Eat foods that are high in color as these contain healthful phytonutrients that can improve your mood and cognitive function.

▶ Eat organic foods whenever they are available. If you are wondering why your food really needs to be organic, check out my "naturally wise women's podcast" Try to avoid foods that may contain hormones, pesticides, herbicides, and food preservatives.

▶ When eating fruits, stick to the whole fruits instead of the juice of the fruit. Whole fruits contain fiber, which is good for your bowels.

▶ Decrease your intake of caffeine and alcohol. It makes your hot flushes worse and messes with your mood.

▶ Eat as many berries as you can. They contain healthful antioxidants, which scavenge for oxygen free radicals and can improve the way your brain works.

▶ Stay away from saturated fats and trans fats, found in processed foods and instead eat healthy fats found in avocados and nuts.

▶ Eat foods that are high in vitamin C, including citrus fruits, red peppers, and spinach. These contain antioxidants that can decrease the dryness of your skin.

▶ Increase the amount of omega 3 fatty acids in your diet. You can find omega 3 fatty acids by eating higher amounts of, flaxseeds, walnuts and brazil nuts for selenium.

▶ I always teach about supplements which are really helpful to manage sleeplessness and anxiety, two of the more important ones are Tryptophan and GABA.

- ► Eat foods high in antioxidant and anti-inflammatory capabilities. You can increase the anti-inflammatory effect by adding turmeric, cayenne pepper, garlic, and rosemary to the foods you eat.

- ► Get more exercise. You can do this by increasing the amount of walking you do, by cycling, swimming, or engaging in any exercise that gets your heart rate going and increases your respiratory rate. Don't exercise like mad when you are already super stressed. Something gentler like yoga or Nia Dance would be much better.

- ► Engage in stress-relieving activities. This can mean enjoying a hobby or taking the time to read a book.

- ► Declutter and simplify your life so you have fewer things to be stressed out over (yes, we are doing this together in the tribe also).

- ► Try this mindfulness meditation or massage therapy, qi gong, yoga, Nia or tai chi to reduce the perception of stress in your life.

- ► Support your adrenal glands by taking vitamins that support the glands. Your adrenal glands also make some reproductive hormones so, if they are supported, you will have fewer symptoms of hot flashes, and night sweats.

Exchange fear for confidence, dread for hopefulness, and uncertainty for excitement as you begin this new, beautiful chapter of your life!

It is my biggest wish for you that you find a way to be a "naturally wise woman", you are the hero of your life story, nobody else is! Please never forget this!

I am on this path, right with you; let me be your guide. I hope we will meet one day!

You've got this! I believe in you!

Love Susanne

Where to find me:
Susanne's website www.susannemcallister.com

Susanne Bio

Susanne McAllister, is an overcomer of a near-death experience at the age of seventeen and a life-long seeker of inner wisdom. A Health and Wellness Coach, Yoga, Nia and Mindfulness Teacher, Hypnotherapist, Psychotherapist and global citizen who believes "that we are all connected". Susanne is the author of several Health and Wellness related books and the host of the "Naturally Wise Women 40+ Podcast". Susanne's passion is working with women to help them to live their best and most authentic lives.

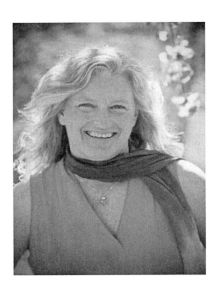

Dr. Maria Maricich

Dr. Maria brings with her an element of surprise. From our very first conversation, I had this mystifying sense that Dr. Maria was way more than what she let on. Yes, we talked about her expertise as a Doctor of Chiropractic and specialized niche in Functional Medicine, but I knew there was more.

Dr. Maria is a beautiful soul who blends into a crowd with quiet reticence. She is a great listener. When Dr. Maria speaks, you better listen.

During her own struggle in menopause, Dr. Maria suffered with brain fog. As a doctor, this was not an option. She had the lives of patients in her care and needed to be on point.

Dr. Maria expanded her expertise to Functional Neurology, looking at the underlying causes of health problems rather than just treating the symptoms.

No wonder I was mystified when I first spoke with her. She is an encyclopedia of conclusive knowledge.

Dr. Maria treats her patients with a pedagogical approach. No patient suffers the same and she invests time in developing their individualized treatment. Dr. Maria is your go-to for all your health care needs.

STOP MENOPAUSE MADNESS, NATURALLY: A BRAIN EXPERT'S PERSPECTIVE

By Dr. Maria Maricich

THE BRAIN IS THE most overlooked aspect of Perimenopause and Menopause. Yet, many of the symptoms such as anxiety, hot flashes, pain, insomnia, and even weight gain originate largely in the brain—not the ovaries. Simply put, the brain becomes inflamed when estrogen levels drop, leading to a myriad of symptoms.

There is a large body of evidence suggesting that the decline in ovarian function as a woman approaches menopause is associated with spontaneous increases in proinflammatory cytokines.[1] Cytokines are chemical messengers in the body which stimulate the immune system, resulting in inflammation.

In general, as we age, health declines. However, statistics show a sharp decline in women's health starting around age forty-five, the average age of perimenopause. Perimenopause is that period of time when hormones are changing and can begin up to ten years prior to the cessation of menstruation. Conditions that increase in risk during this time period are cardiovascular disease, osteoporosis, dementia and Alzheimer's disease, arthritis and autoimmune disease. The one thing all these diseases have in common is inflammation.

In this chapter we cover exactly what happens in the brain with this increase of inflammation, why many of the challenges women are facing appear during the perimenopause phase, and what to do to resolve these issues so you can live exceptionally happy and healthy now and for many years to come.

The name of the game for menopausal symptoms that are brain related is Neuroinflammation. Neuroinflammation is a result of the increased cytokine activity which happens suddenly when sex hormone levels decline. There are three main effects of Neuroinflammation we will cover: first the influence on neurotransmitters, second the upset of the emotional brain, and third the impact on the gut-brain axis.

Hormone replacement therapy, whether bioidentical or not, does not typically reverse neuroinflammation once it has begun. Of the thirty or more symptoms related to menopause, only a few are solely due to hormone loss and not due to the resulting inflammation. Furthermore, when the inflammatory cytokine system becomes overactivated during perimenopause, it often remains overactivated well beyond the menopausal years—whether or not there has been hormone replacement.[2]

Neurotransmitters

Neurotransmitters are chemical messengers in the brain. They cause neurons to fire. When neurotransmitters are unable to do their job well, we see all kinds of brain-related symptoms. The most commonly understood neurotransmitter is serotonin as it is linked with depression. But several other neurotransmitters are necessary for a high-functioning brain as well.

Neurotransmitters play a role in our moods, memory, learning, self-esteem, anxiety, motivation, and energy levels. They affect how we perceive ourselves and the world around us. We must have excellent neurotransmitter function in order to have good mental health.

The surplus of cytokines floating around in the brain during perimenopause compete with neurotransmitters, causing a reduction of neurotransmitter activity. This explains the appearance of poor moods, fatigue, and insomnia.

The Emotional Brain

The same cytokines and resulting neuroinflammation have an effect on the limbic area of the brain, also known as the emotional brain. In neuroscience we call it plasticity when the brain changes itself in response to changes in the body. The limbic brain gets ramped up with inflammation, causing more stress in this area—and more plasticity. The limbic brain gets overloaded and we are left with a short fuse, feeling irritable or emotionally up and down. Many women will be confused by their lack of control over their emotions.

The Autonomic Nervous System—that part of the nervous system that regulates all the organs and glands without us having to think about it—has centers within the limbic area. It too gets ramped up and therefore stressed. When the Autonomic System is stressed it becomes imbalanced and shuts down the activity of digestion. Sudden digestive issues can emerge. The increased stress can also trigger increased blood pressure, heart-related symptoms, and headaches.

Stress affecting the Autonomic Nervous System causes a release of the stress hormone, cortisol. Cortisol in excess induces fat storage, especially around the middle—hence the weight gain that is common in perimenopause. Cortisol also kills brain cells, especially in the memory centers of the brain.

Gut-Brain Axis

The gut-brain axis is a bidirectional communication between the gut and the central nervous system. Numerous studies show that the health of the gut has a profound effect on brain function and emotions. We have already seen that digestion can be disrupted during perimenopause. What's more, the increased cytokine activity causes a breakdown of the intestinal barrier, also known as leaky gut. The lining of the intestinal tract becomes more porous, allowing the good bacteria in the gut to "leak" into the blood, triggering the immune response to release more cytokines further winding up the whole neuro-endocrine-immune system.[3]

Frequently when there is leaky gut, biochemicals are released that cause leaky brain. Leaky brain means molecules that should not enter the brain such as toxins and bacteria are now able to enter, again instigating more neuroinflammation. Cyrex Labs offers blood tests that can help determine if either of these conditions are happening.

Women are twice as likely as men to get Alzheimer's and dementia. We know that inflammation is the biggest risk factor for these devastating diseases. It is this sudden wind of inflammation affecting the brain that makes a woman more susceptible to neurodegenerative diseases.

Unwinding Neuroinflammation

Toxins, viruses, parasites, bacteria, teeth problems, gut problems, anemia, poor blood sugar regulation, the standard American (inflammatory) diet, stress, food sensitivities, and poor sleep habits can all provoke inflammation. Most people have some degree of inflammation in the body. Estrogen keeps the inflammation calm, like a wet forest. But when estrogen diminishes it's as though the forest dries up and the flames take off, potentially affecting many tissues, especially the brain.

In order to restore balance, we must address all the sources of inflammation. Following are steps to squelch the inflammation:

1. **Anti-inflammatory diet**. Diet is the foundation of reducing inflammation in the body and the brain. Gluten, dairy, egg, soy, corn, peanuts, tomatoes, caffeine, alcohol, trans fats and sugar are the most inflammatory items to consume, even if you are not allergic to them. Try eliminating them for 30 days. Here is the perfect program to guide you step by step in reducing an overactive immune system, or try a ketogenic diet.

2. **Remove toxins.** Toxins keep the body inflamed. Reduce your exposure to toxins by eating only organic foods. Be sure to include lots of fresh produce to facilitate flushing of toxins. Use cleaning products that are environmentally friendly. Get an air purifier. New research shows a link between plastics and autoimmunity to the brain, so try to remove plastic from your life.[4]

3. **Do a comprehensive detox program.** Over time the body can accumulate unneeded hormones, plastics, herbicides and pesticides, molds, and other environmental contaminants.

It is nearly impossible to avoid toxins in today's world. Each of the above toxins can disrupt hormone function and increase the inflammatory response. However, removing them is not always an easy task. If done improperly, toxins can be freed from other tissues only to end up in the brain, causing more problems.

A proper and effective detox program will have herbs to support the organs of detoxification including the liver, kidneys, and lymphatics. It will also have nutraceuticals to support release of toxins at a cellular level. And finally, it will have a binder to be sure the toxins are bound and released from the body rather than left free-floating in the body to cause further damage.

Addressing environmental contaminants and toxins promotes overall health and is recommended for all ages. Click here for a link to my favorite detox system. This program is a combined gut-repair and detox program that everybody could benefit from.

4. **Repair your gut.** Repairing leaky gut will also help repair leaky brain. The process requires following a restricted diet, taking nutritional compounds that help reduce intestinal inflammation and repair the intestinal lining (see below), and taking probiotics to help balance gut bacteria populations. Digestive enzymes are beneficial too.

   The diet includes lots of organic vegetables, quality meats, fish and chicken, fermented foods, and good fats such as coconut, olive, and avocado oil. Foods to eliminate include all grains, nuts and seeds, nightshades, eggs, soy corn, legumes, and alcohol. More information can be found here.

5. **Balance blood sugar.** The main fuel for the brain is glucose, also known as blood sugar. A drop or rise in blood sugar can trigger an immediate hot flash and further perpetuate the inflammatory cascade. Supporting blood sugar is critical for improving menopausal symptoms, improving brain health, and for recovery from any type of inflammation.

Unstable blood sugar is linked with many of the symptoms of menopause including brain fog, depression, coping skills, and insomnia. Blood sugar balance is necessary for balanced brain chemistry and prevention of neurodegeneration.

To balance blood sugar, eliminate sugar, sweets, and caffeine from your diet. Reduce overall intake of carbohydrates, replacing them with organic produce, proteins, and quality fats. And never let yourself get too hungry. If you are having trouble kicking the sugar habit, try this program.

6. **Exercise.** Exercise gets oxygen to the brain, helps blood sugar balance, and stimulates nerve growth factors. Even if you don't have time to go to the gym or get out for a hike, do something to get your heart rate up. Raising your heart rate up, even for one minute, helps brain function. I love the 7-minute workout app for this. You can find it for both android and apple phones.

   Over-exercising can be a problem for the brain—just like under-exercising. If you feel fatigued and have a hard time recovering from exercise, it is a sign your body is not able to handle that level of exercise, due to depleted cellular energy. In this case, you must first implement some of the other tools provided here to regain balance. Over-exercising can cause more inflammation. For women who are exercising a lot but still can't lose weight, this may be the cause.

7. **My Favorite Supplements.**

   a. Turmeric, or more specifically, curcuminoids in doses of 500mg or more, will calm cytokine activity.

   b. Short Chain Fatty Acids such as butyrate, propionate, and acetate feed the lining of the intestine and calm inflammation in the brain.

   c. Resveratrol is a polyphenol that restores balance in the gut and reduces overall inflammation.

   d. Vitamin D is an immune modulator, helps the gut, and has been shown to reduce the risk of seventeen different cancers.

e. Glutathione helps combat the damage done by inflammation and supports healthy liver function.

f. Milk thistle is a liver support herb, helping to clear toxins and balance hormones.

8. **Sleep.** Do everything you can to get a good night's sleep. Sleep helps the brain repair, helps with weight concerns, and so much more.[5] All the steps above can help with sleep. In addition, turn off all screens (TV, computer) an hour before bed, use calming essential oils like lavender, go to bed by ten o'clock, and listen to sleep-inducing meditations (there are lots on YouTube or in the app store).

How I Became Interested in Easing the Menopause Experience

A while back, I was sitting in a hotel conference room with a large group of doctors, many of whom were younger than me. It was January, so it was cold out and I had on lots of layers. I was there for a workshop on how to take a successful health practice to the online world. I was really excited for this workshop because I was ready to expand the reach of my practice. About half an hour in, I get hit with a hot flash, so I'm subtly trying to take off layers, starting with the scarf I had wrapped around my neck, then my jacket, then putting my hair up in a ponytail. Fifteen minutes later, I'm doing it all in reverse. I continued this ritual approximately every hour for the next two days, trying not to be conspicuous.

We go a couple more hours, and I'm getting more and more enthused about what I'm learning. Then it's time to break out into groups and mastermind what we've learned. I feel like the third wheel, there doesn't seem to be anybody who wants to partner with me. Then at the cocktail party that evening I'm feeling shunned in conversations. People seem to be ignoring me and turning a cold shoulder. The same thing happens the next day. I go to bed thinking this has been a weird weekend—I'm not used to being treated like this. In High School I was popular and through my adult life I've never had a hard time getting attention. I'm an Olympian (1984 Alpine Downhill Skiing) so people often want to chat about that. I've been to tons of professional seminars in my career and never have I felt invisible before. Then it dawned on me, and this is what I wrote in my journal when I got home:

I'm 58 years old. I'm 20 lbs. overweight. I don't believe in coloring my hair and I can't be bothered with painting my face every morning just so I look a little more attractive. I just want to be me and I guess that me is not the "hottie" I used to be. I wanted to shout out "Don't you know I'm an Olympian? Don't you know I'm a well-respected doctor in my community? Don't you know I graduated Magna Cum Laude from the same school you went to? Don't you know my generation of doctors paved the way so you younger ones could make a bigger difference? Don't you know I'm a worthy human being too?"

I realized that not only do women have to deal with all kinds of health concerns, but the culture treats them with less respect—or might we say disrespect?

I was already helping women with hormone issues, but from that day forward I made it my mission to empower women to be their best self, physically, emotionally, socially, and spiritually through menopause and beyond. The principles I've shared with you here are meant to do just that.

I have prepared a Free Checklist to help you determine what areas to address first.

Bio Dr. Maria Maricich

Being interested in natural health and maximizing human potential from an early age as part of her journey to the Olympics in 1984, it's only logical that Dr. Maria would bring that into her professional career. Dr. Maria Maricich is the founder of The Wellness Clinic in Sun Valley, Idaho and Dr. Maria Online, a virtual practice. She is a Doctor of Chiropractic and specializes in the new and emerging fields of Functional Medicine and Functional Neurology, which look for underlying causes of health problems rather than just treating the symptoms. Her passion is understanding the mechanisms of the brain and applying evidence-based natural methods to improve function; from moods to memory to anti-aging. With this understanding, she recognizes that the brain is the most overlooked influencer during the perimenopause/menopause phase and has been able to adapt her methods to help women overcome the more common symptoms such as anxiety, insomnia, pain, hot flashes, and fatigue. She can be found at www.DrMariaMaricich.com or https://www.facebook.com/DrMariaOnline.

References

1. https://www.ncbi.nlm.nih.gov/pubmed/11844745
2. https://www.ncbi.nlm.nih.gov/pubmed/7789055
3. https://www.ncbi.nlm.nih.gov/pmc/articles/PMC5581153/
4. https://www.ncbi.nlm.nih.gov/pubmed/27610592
5. https://www.ncbi.nlm.nih.gov/pubmed/31287027

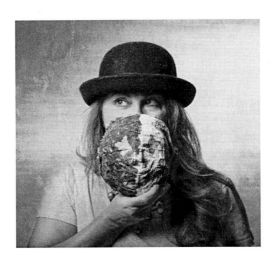

Anjl Rodee

She's the highlight of my day (by her own admission) and will be yours too, when you get to know her.

As a professional musician, comedian and artist, yes, all of those, Anjl has you feeling great just by being in her presence.

A humble, jovial, passionate, generous, tenderhearted, adventurous and loving woman, I knew I had to know her from the moment I walked into the painting class she was teaching,

She is quick witted and will have you belly laughing until it hurts. Anjl has an uncanny way of making you feel like you're a gifted musician, comedian or artist by encouraging you in your creativity. She will help you open the box of creative expression and take you into a realm that ignites your own personal passions. She's someone you need to know too.

MOD PODGE AND MENOPAUSE: CREATIVITY IS THE ANSWER. WHAT WAS THE QUESTION?

By Anjl Rodee

MY SIBLINGS AND I USED to play something we called Celebrity Hotel. We'd choose a famous group or family; The Osmonds, Jackson 5, Partridge Family and the Monkees were in top rotation. As the oldest, I always got the choicest character, and usually nabbed the lead singer role; Donny, Michael, Keith and Davey Jones. We'd be on tour, see, and when checking into the hotel, we'd realize we'd forgotten our wallets and would need to put on a free show at the hotel to cover the cost of our rooms. We'd put on our favorite vinyl record and sing and dance away the afternoon.

Kids love to play make believe. They mimic parents and heroes, trying on all sorts of idyllic careers for size. They pretend to be teachers and astronauts, parents and veterinarians.

We are born creative, and when we are young, we have a lot of fun with it. We sing at the top of our lungs everywhere, not just the car or shower–we dance like we just won the lottery; we draw and paint with equal parts joy and intensity.

Somewhere along the line, however, we are discouraged away from these artistic endeavors that give us so much joy. Unfortunately, our society has taken these self-expressions of creativity- singing, dancing, writing and painting- and quantified them right out of daily existence for most people. If you're not good at them, you shouldn't do them. Or worse–if you are good at them, you still shouldn't waste your time developing that skill, as you'll only end up a starving artist.

I am an artist. I've always been an artist. In the second grade, I was famous for my spot-on drawings of Snoopy. I won a statewide poster design contest in the 4th grade, and I was the only 8th grader invited to a summer art camp for high schoolers put on by the University of Wisconsin.

I am a creative person. And you? You are also a creative person! We all are. Creativity is a uniquely human trait. When we think of the 'Creative', we think of people like Mozart and Picasso and Steve Jobs. It's great that they are in the world, able to make a living by sharing the fruits of their creative output with the rest of us.

But creativity isn't just relegated to the super talented. Studies show that we all have the same 'building blocks of creativity' that artistic geniuses do!

It's the thing that makes us inherently human; our ability to create. We are all creative beings. The ability to imagine and then make things is our most primordial purpose. And not just because we need to fill that empty space on the living room wall; creative endeavors are actually good for you, in a multitude of ways.

You are not destined to suffer from mental and emotional decline! Our brains do something wonderful at menopause- they stay in a state of perpetual creativity. When your period stops, your hormones don't experience the same surges and cycles. Women report better creativity after menopause than when they were younger.

We find ourselves perfectly honed for a creative power surge! We fear failure less. We overflow with inspiration. We have a lifetime of experiences, visions and stories, just waiting to come out.

Medical research shows that creative activities affect both the brain and body, leading to benefits like increased mood, decreased anxiety, heightened cognitive function, reduced risk of chronic illnesses and improved immune health.

One of the most obvious benefits of having a creative practice is that it's a way to elevate mood. If you were to ask most people why they pursue a creative hobby or outlet, they'd likely respond with something like "it makes me feel good". Many people may not understand fully why their creative expression makes them feel good, they just know that it's something they must look forward to outside their normal routine. For those of you that like the idea of meditating but have a hard time focusing on not focusing (pointing fingers at myself), painting and sketching reaps the same benefits as meditation, and you end up with cool stuff to hang on your fridge when you're done. Win-win!!

Creative activities that you enjoy are fulfilling and uplifting. It's something you can turn to if you've had a bad day and use to release and express yourself. Doing a creative thing that you feel good about contributes to building a positive self-identity. As you commit yourself to a kind of art, whether it be writing, music, painting, or just taking interesting photos with your phone, you're demonstrating to yourself that you can develop a skill over time, which is an important component of self-esteem. Do not listen to that inner voice that harps 'you're not an artist/singer/dancer.' OH YES YOU ARE!! If paint has hit the canvas, you're an artist! If sound is coming out any of your head holes, you are singing! If your arms and/or legs are moving, you're a dancer!

In addition to bettering mood, creative expression can also be healing for those suffering from anxiety and depression. Research has found that music therapy and theatre are great methods for decreasing anxiety. One of the suggested reasons for this is that music calms brain activity, leading to a sense of emotional balance.

Another excellent way to combat anxiety and depression is laughter. We'll save that chat for another chapter, but by all means in the meantime, rent yourself a funny movie or take your BFF to a local improv theatre. Nothing lifts a heavy mind or heart like laughter.

Having a creative outlet has positive impacts on cognitive health. Researchers have found evidence as to how creativity affects the brain. Musicians, in particular, have been studied for the heightened connectivity between their left and right brain hemispheres. This is believed to be one of the reasons why Einstein was a genius—his mastery of the violin allowed him to effectively use both sides of his brain simultaneously. Just an hour and a half of creative practice every week will drastically improve cognitive function. That's 12 minutes a day! Working on something creative, whether it's writing a short story or working on a paint-by-number of your favorite masterpiece, helps apply problem-solving and critical thinking skills as well. Other forms of creative expression such as karaoke, open mics and improv comedy, have shown to help older adults maintain cognitive skills.

There are many creatives who reached their heights well into midlife - Frida Kahlo, Jane Lynch, Picasso and Vera Wang, to name a few. While doing creative things won't outright cure disease or block menopausal symptoms, it surely can and will take focus away from pain and discomfort. Like when you have a headache, then you stub your toe and forget that your head hurts! Filling in coloring book pages is a whole lot more pleasant than that scenario.

Getting creative doesn't have to mean turning your guest room into a crafting palace or sinking your savings into singing lessons (unless that's what you want to do). Here are a few ways to get your creative juices flowing. Find something that sparks excitement and joy, and dive in!

1. Go for a walk.
   This is a great place to start. Just walk and stay present in each moment. Observe the sights, sounds and smells around you. Where does your mind go? Could you write a description about your surroundings; capture it with paint, sing a song about it, or take a photograph? Follow this instinct and see where it might lead.

2. Interview your inner child.
   Or the child that was you, before you were you. Did you love art class or choir in middle school? Is there an unfinished novel in the bottom drawer of your desk? Was making up dances with your friends something that gave you joy? Rekindle your love for these things. What a great way to get back in touch with your best you!

3. Learn how to knit.
   Knitting is SO good. It's kind of like a creative green superfood (whatever that is. There is probably a chapter about it

somewhere else in this book). Knitting is the new yoga! There are now studies proving that the rhythmic act of knitting offers benefits similar to meditation. It reduces stress levels and blood pressure. It also stimulates the logical parts of your brain, strengthening concentration skills and even the immune system.

4. Attend a paint and sip.
   Paint and sip parties, where an art instructor guides you in making your own masterpiece, are a fun and social way to get creative. And have a relaxing glass of wine or three to boot! In one study, participants who knocked back an average of three drinks were more creative than people who didn't drink at all. Just saying.

5. Take creativity to the kitchen.
   Experiment with new recipes or try a cuisine you've never cooked before. Visit a farmer's market or specialty store and buy ingredients that are unusual or unfamiliar to you to use as the basis for an adventurous meal.

6. Attend a creative event.
   Even small towns have poetry readings, open mic nights, book signings, recitals, craft fairs and art shows. When I need inspiration, I know I'll find it when watching creative people doing creative things.

7. Sing, sing, and sing some more.
   Singing is another creative superfood, in my opinion. It releases endorphins that improve your mood and give you a natural high. It also releases oxytocin, which has been found to alleviate anxiety and stress. Singing exercises your lungs and diaphragm. Memorizing lyrics encourages better concentration skills. It involves multiple senses, which increase brain function in general. Do it everywhere. The world will thank you for it.

8. Give rap a chance.
   Want to up your concentration game even further? Make up a rap song about your buddy Joe (any one syllable name will do).

"I know a guy; his name is Joe. He can't run fast, he's really slow. Yesterday he stubbed is toe. He loves Edgar Allen Poe." Same benefits as singing; also, your grandkids will think you are the COOLEST!

9. Make yourself a portable creativity kit.
    Take a smallish bag and fill it with things like a small notebook and fun pens. Then when you're waiting for an oil change or root canal, instead of phone scrolling, you can doodle and sketch and write. It will help move your mind from 'I can't' and place it firmly in the joy of creating.

10. Have a dance party.
    I'm not going to lie, this one is the hardest for me. That's not easy for me to admit, as a former ballroom dance instructor, but there it is... I'm not comfortable dancing, even in the privacy of my own home. But here's the thing - there is no faster way to boost happiness, foster self-expression, maximize brain function, and just all out have fun and it's fairly instantaneous. No supplies to purchase, no waiting 'til the paint dries.

For more ideas on how to be creative, visit me here: www. modmeno.com.

I've recently become aware of the term PMZ - Post Menopausal Zest. It's not a stripy soap, and it's not garnish for a craft cocktail. PMZ is the burst of energy, creativity and lust for life (and other things) that shows up after the throngs of menopause die down.

That's the light at the end of the tunnel. That's the good news, but you don't have to wait for the PMZ train to roll into town to feel better. Singing in the car, dancing like no one is watching and crafting bad poetry with refrigerator magnets can improve your quality of life. So, don't wait until you're on tour without your wallet! Grab that hairbrush, crank some Beyoncé and put on a show that your mirror will never forget.

Bio

Anjl Rodee wears a lot of hats. Celebrity artist, improv comedian, and working musician; with more chapeaus on the rack, so to speak.

Anjl is the founder of BrushCapades, using entertainment to encourage the creativity, meditative essence, and joy of painting. She is building a community of people that enjoy the positive energy of a creative lifestyle. She believes that you shouldn't paint because you are good at it, but because it is good for you.

Anjl is an improv comedian, currently enjoying a committed nine-year relationship with ComedySportz.

Anjl is co-creator of Dear Anjl and Marilynn, an online humor column where relationship advice is doled out with salt and wit.

She is working on her first book *A is for Aneurism*.

Follow Anjl on Instagram https://www.instagram.com/anjlkr/
Friend Anjl on Facebook https://www.facebook.com/anjlr
Make art with Anjl at https://www.modmeno.com
See all the other creative stuff Anjl does at https://www.anjlrodee.com

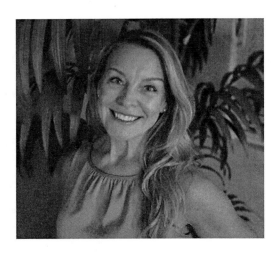

Sandy Hartwell

Sandy is the epitome of success. Raising her son as a single mother, she exemplifies dedication and resolve in building her global business, Heart-Well Fitness and Health Coaching for women.

When Sandy called me and we talked, I was enthralled by her tender demeanor. I could immediately sense her authentic desire to revolutionize the lives of women in menopause. Sandy has developed her life-changing regimen from her own place of pain.

Whether she is providing healthy yet decadent meal plans, giving her health tip of the day, demonstrating the ease of exercise in your own home, encouraging you to embrace the beauty of the outdoors or simply take a deep breath, you will know you've made a friend for life who will lovingly walk beside you.

She is a sympathetic, softhearted, patient, intuitive, relentless, enduring friend. Sandy is THE ONLY health and fitness coach you will ever need.

FOOD AND FITNESS IN MENOPAUSE: SIMPLE HABITS TO REDUCE SYMPTOMS AND ACHIEVE OPTIMAL HEALTH

By Sandy Hartwell

OUR BODIES, IN ANY stage of menopause, sometimes feel out of control. This transition is often uncomfortable, even scary at times. Hot flashes, night sweats, weight gain, brain fog, mood swings, lower libido, lack of energy, these are common complaints. I'm not going to tell you that you can fix it, but I will share ideas regarding nutrition, movement and self-care that can help you understand, appreciate and embrace change so you can be more comfortable, less afraid and more confident.

In midlife, our bodies are supposed to change. There are usually good reasons for it doing the things it does. The more we fight these natural changes, the harder our body works to adapt, which is why resistance is often futile. Let's take, for example, that extra body fat we are storing in places we didn't store fat before.

In midlife, our estradiol (a type of estrogen) production shuts down and our body relies partially on adipose (a type of fat) tissue to produce similar hormones. While a certain amount of fat on our body is necessary for hormonal health, too much fat increases our risk of metabolic diseases and cancers that are estrogen dominant, like breast cancer and ovarian cancer. If you're unsure if your body fat percentage is too high or too low, check your body composition. Many household scales can now give you a pretty good approximation within 3%. Studies suggest that a healthy body fat percentage for women 40-60 years of age is 23-35%.

These hormone changes can also lead to a change in our shape. Our lean body mass (muscle, bone and connective tissue) decreases as body fat increases. This is called sarcopenia and quality nutrition and exercise can help, as can Hormone Replacement Therapy (HRT) if you decide with your doctor to go that route.

Food and Quality Nutrition

Regardless of your Body Fat Percentage, adopting a quality nutrition program has many benefits. It's not just for weight loss. A good quality nutrition program has been shown to increase energy, improve mood, reduce hot flashes and bloat, and improve sleep quality due to reduction in sugar. Additionally, what you eat will affect your muscle strength, bone density, blood-sugar, cholesterol, risk of cardio-vascular disease and inflammatory diseases.

Good hydration can help with dizziness or vertigo, it improves skin, hair and nails, aids in digestion and helps minimize water retention. Limiting alcohol consumption may also help increase hydration as well as reduce mood swings, brain fog, weight gain and pain associated with inflammation.

Eat whole foods or foods that are minimally processed. How do you know if it's a whole food? If it ran, swam, flew or grew, it's a whole food. If you can dig it out of the ground, pick it off a tree or bush it's a whole food. Basically, if you would recognize it in nature, it's a whole food (think chicken leg = yes, chicken sausage = no).

Minimally processed foods are those that still have less than three ingredients like ground beef, canned tomatoes, nut butters, some oils (avocado, coconut, olive).

Prioritize quality nutrition. Fresh fruits and vegetables, which are high in antioxidants many help with inflammation, bloat and increase energy. For hot flashes, try omega-3 rich flax seeds, foods that are phytoestrogenic like soy (tempeh, fresh edamame, tofu).

Any sustainable nutrition program must be easy, enjoyable and the foods must aid in attaining your goal if it is to be adopted as a lifestyle change. For this reason, I always start my clients with this easy to use, take it anywhere, Hand Portion Control Guide www. HandPortions.com. It's convenient because you take, your hands with you wherever you go, work lunches, restaurants, social gatherings and family dinners. Hands are scaled to your own body, so it provides reasonable amounts of nutrient dense foods, preventing deficiencies. This guide will help you meet your macro-nutrient needs for protein, fats, vegetables, carbohydrates and caloric needs without having to weigh, measure or count calories.

Keep in mind that protein needs go up as we age. Increasing protein means more lean muscle and increased bone density especially if you're doing resistance training.

Read nutrition labels. Quality nutrition can certainly ease or alleviate discomfort by improving digestion, decreasing disease risk, reducing inflammation, improving skin quality and promoting dental health.

Become a food detective by turning the package over to see the nutrition label and the ingredients.

If you can't pronounce, don't eat it.

If you wouldn't recognize it in nature, don't eat it.

Avoid genetically modified foods (GMO).

Look for sugars. Most words ending with "ose" (fructose, sucrose, etc.) are added sugars. The American Heart Association recommends women should consume no more than 100 calories (25g) of added sugar per day.

Fitness/Regular Exercise That You Truly Enjoy

We know you can't outrun a bad diet, and that the eat less, exercise more approach won't work anymore because as our hormone production decreases, our need for recovery and stress reduction increases, and both eating less and exercising more are stressors to our bodies.

In my research of the hundreds of women I've worked with over the past fifteen years, I have discovered that sweet spot for women and the good news is you can be fit over forty, fifty, sixty and beyond.

The sooner you begin, the more you will benefit. The health risks of not exercising are certainly worth getting out of your comfort zone for. Here are a few:

▶ *Decline in cardio/vascular health (heart disease, circulation and blood pressure)*

▶ *Continue to gain weight and exacerbate depression and irritability*

▶ *Muscle degeneration and loose skin*

▶ *Morning stiffness particularly in the back and neck*

▶ *Increased risk of metabolic syndrome and diabetes*

The good news is, it's never too late to start and the many benefits of regular exercise include:

▶ *decreased fat storage*

▶ *improved insulin sensitivity*

▶ *improved mood and sleep*

▶ *increased bone density and strength*

▶ *improved circulation and blood pressure*

▶ *improved strength and coordination*

Now you may have less time now to exercise but don't let that stop you. Do what you can and know that something is ALWAYS better than nothing. If you have a base level of fitness, try 10-20-minutes of high intensity interval training (HIIT). This approach to training is just the right balance of resistance training exercises combined with bouts of getting your heart rate up with some high intensity cardio movements. Keeping in mind that not everyone has access to a gym, so I created my NEXT LEVEL FITNESS workouts using body weight to build strength.

If you're just starting out, good for you! What's important is to be consistent and start where you are. Gentle Yoga may be good for women starting from sedentary. For weight bearing movement and resistance training, hire a personal trainer who understands how to train a woman's body at midlife. In my BASE LEVEL FITNESS program this is the exact approach I use as an introduction to exercise.

Mind/Body Connection

Let's face it. Women are nurturers by nature. We are the cheerleaders of our tribe whether it be encouraging our children, praising significant others, coworkers, or lending an optimistic ear to a friend. We have nurtured our children, our businesses and in many instances our aging parents, sometimes simultaneously and often, at the expense of ourselves.

I can recall countless conversations with women who have come in for consultation and echo some version of "I don't know what *I* like, anymore. I'm unable to do many of the things I used to do, and I don't have anyone to talk to about it." Often, they feel hopeless, sitting with some new version themselves that has taken a back seat to the burdensome responsibilities they so dutifully signed up for. Unfortunately, they often feel resentful toward those they have loved and served and feel alone and ashamed of how they look and feel.

Hot flashes, weight gain, mood swings and brain fog, loss of libido and vaginal dryness, not to mention hair loss AND growth in the all the wrong places. REALLY? No wonder we don't want to talk about it! The more discouraged we become, we find ourselves feeling lonely, scared, confused and hopeless. Like we've lost our spark. Understand that there is much we **can** do to improve how we experience this transition and it begins with a mind-set shift. You can start by practicing a little self-compassion. That's right. Less self-sabotage and more self-love. Talk to yourself the way you would speak to a friend who's struggling. Be nice.

Bio Sandy Hartwell

Having grown up working in the family garden, snacking from Grandfather's blueberry bushes and rhubarb garden, helping Mom bake bread from scratch each week and spending school vacations learning to cook in grandmother's kitchen, it's no wonder Sandy found her passion in sharing her whole foods approach with women as a natural career path. Sandy is the owner of Heart-well Fitness and Health Coaching and the creator of The Next Level

Living Club, a virtual classroom and online support community for health-minded women. She is a Certified Personal Trainer, Health and Nutrition Coach specializing in women's health, specifically through the stages of perimenopause, menopause and post menopause. Her passion is understanding what a woman goes through physically, mentally and spiritually during this midlife transition, and applying clean eating, daily movement and self-care to make the experience a celebration. When a girl starts menses it's a celebration of womanhood, when a woman carries and delivers a child it's a celebration of life. Why then, when a woman matures and her ovaries naturally slow the production of estrogen, is our response to this process one of shame, fear, sorrow and pain resulting in a silent suffering? Our bodies are supposed to change, but we don't have to fight it. Through her teachings on simple lifestyle changes, incorporating whole foods, daily movement and nurturing self-care habits, her clients can reconnect the mind with the body, build confidence and apply the tools necessary to stop researching and start living!

Reach out to Sandy personally at:

Sandy@heartwellfitness.com
www.heartwellfitness.com
Follow her on Facebook at: https://www.facebook.com/
HeartWellFitness/
Join her private online community for health-minded women at:
https://www.facebook.com/groups/NextLevelLivingClub/

To learn more about her programs for menopausal women, visit www.NextLevelLivingClub.com.

Tips on improving the quality of your nutrition:

▶ *Start drinking more water. Ideally, aim for half your bodyweight in ounces of water, but if you're not used to drinking water or you're a soda drinker, start with what's manageable. Replace one a day with an 8 oz glass of water and gradually decrease soda and increase water until you achieve your goal. If you want to add a bit of flavor, try a twist or a squeeze of lemon or lime.*

► *Limit caffeine, sugar and alcohol, especially in the afternoon and evening for improved sleep, decreased night sweats and hot flashes*

► *Assuming your active each day and eat about three meals and a snack each day, for each meal, women might begin by eating:*

  o *1 palm size portion of protein dense food (lean chicken, eggs, fish, beans, lentils)*

  o *2 fist size portions of vegetables (eat a rainbow of colorful fruits and vegetables)*

  o *1 cupped handful of carbohydrate dense food (rice, potato, sweet potato, quinoa)*

  o *1 thumb size portion of fat dense food (nuts, nut butter, avocado, olive oil, avocado or coconut oil)*

Tips on incorporating movement and exercise:

► *Warming up your joints prior to exercising with yoga or 5 minute of mobility exercises will help prevent exercise induced injury and keep joints lubricated and flexible.*

► *Moving at a moderate intensity 2-4 times per week for 30-60 minutes per session may help with cramps often associated with changing menstrual cycles and inflammation. Most people can participate in walking or moving in the water or gentle yoga.*

► *Weight bearing movement or resistance training 2-3 times a week will improve bone density and strength as well as keep your muscles strong and flexible. Hire a personal trainer to help with this if you're just starting out.*

► *Recover 1-2 days a week. Exercise is, after all a stressor on the body. Recovery reduces cortisol (a hormone known to increase appetite resulting in weight gain). A casual walk at an easy, conversational pace is an effective way to keep moving while reducing stress. Aim for a balance between work and recovery.*

How to improve your Mind/Body Connection

► *Eat slowly and mindfully. Put your fork down and sip water between bites. Aim for 20-minute meals. Notice the color, aroma, flavor and texture of your food. Enjoy each bite. You will reduce cravings later and reduce the amount of food you consume at each meal when you are mindful of the experience. Use the convenient portion control guide under nutrition tips in this chapter.*

► *Sleep 7-9 hours a night. Use quality nutrition to reduce night sweats and insomnia. Experiment with natural sleep remedies like valerian root, tart cherry juice and isoflavones (from soy).*

► *Go for a leisurely walk in nature. Aim for 30-60 minutes daily or a minimum of three times a week. On these walks take some deep breathes, notice the sights and smells along your path, appreciate your surroundings. When done consistently, this can lower stress and cortisol (stress hormones) considerably, making way for a more positive mindset, an increase in patience with yourself and others, tolerance and improves sleep quality.*

► *Listen to your body for Hunger Cues. Eat when you feel hungry and stop eating before your full. If you combine this with mindful eating, you'll notice that at some point before all your food is gone, you are not hungry anymore. This is the time to stop. It will keep you from feeling sleepy after a meal, even out your energy for the rest of the day and reduce the number of calories you consume at each meal.*

CHOICE is the most powerful tool we have. Everything boils down to choice. We exist in a field of infinite possibilities. Every choice we make shuts an infinite number of doors and opens an infinite number of doors. At any point, we can change the direction of our lives by a simple choice.

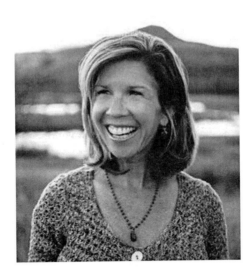

Julie Zolfo

I met Julie on a hike, traversing the arduous slopes of the Cascades in Central Oregon. I knew she was someone I needed to know.

Julie is the personification of endurance. After losing her job in corporate America, she broached this unforeseen opportunity and chose to aggressively pursue her passions, not without struggles, of course. Without fully understanding what this looked like for her, she became a student of change.

As the days and years ensued, Julie ultimately became a master educator, teaching women how to tap into their passions and pursue what brings fulfillment. She practices what she teaches. She is a life enhancer and destination changer.

No wonder I felt like I needed her in my life. She has become a dear friend, a friend who is steadfast and consistent, generous with her knowledge and skills, empathetic in conversation and loyal to the core. Julie will lead you from crisis to empowerment.

THE MENOPAUSAL MAP: HOW ASTROLOGY SHINED A LIGHT ON MY DARKEST (AND HOTTEST) NIGHTS

By Julie Zolfo

"CONGRATULATIONS! YOU'RE A WOMAN now. What a wonderful Christmas gift." These were the so-called words of comfort and wisdom my mom offered as I laid in my bed on Christmas Day in a fetal position, combating the nonstop onslaught of excruciating abdominal cramps in my sweat soaked new Christmas pajamas.

What was so celebratory about this moment of pain, perspiration and profuse blood pouring out of my vagina? Was this really going to be my new life, every month, for the next forty to fifty years? Thankfully at age 12 I had been educated in school and by my parents about the "normal" physical and emotional changes happening to my body yet getting my period for the first time was still scary, overwhelming and most of all, embarrassing.

From "Aunt Flow" to "The Curse" I learned quickly countless ways to talk about my period with girlfriends without ever saying the word period. It never occurred to me, back then, how a new generation of young women, like me, were being conditioned by a previous generation of women to repeat the unhealthy cycle of not talking openly about a critical life milestone. If getting our period was so natural, why was it so taboo to talk about it without using code words?

Fast forward thirty-five years, I started to hear a slew of different code words whispered among my girlfriends, this time to describe their irregular periods, night sweats, brain fog or their periods stopped completely. Was I back here again in the dark ages of unhealthy secrets to deal with my next life changes?

Ironically, it was about this time, age forty-six, I remember experiencing a very awkward menopause moment. In front of my dad and my older sister I tried to skirt around a hot flash I was having.

"What?" I said with a smile, redirecting my question back to my sister.

"Is everything alright? You just got up to go stand in an open doorway when its forty something degrees outside. For someone who always complains of being cold, you're acting odd."

This was a key deciding moment. Do I continue to play coy, downplaying what was going on within my body or was I going to just own it, without shame?

Jokingly I replied, "I experiencing a Hawaiian volcano erupting within me while simultaneously talking to you." I giggled. Neither my sister nor Dad laughed along. I was going to need to clarify specifically what was happening.

"Let me say it another way...

"I was experiencing the worse hot flash ever."

There I said it! I didn't care what their reaction was. I was done making others feel comfortable at the expense of my own discomfort. This madness of secrets and shame needed to stop.

Later that night I called my seventy-year-old mom in Florida. I needed to hear what she experienced during "the change" in her life. Unlike the educational classes provided in middle school about menstruation, I had no access to understanding the stages of menopause or mid-life happenings in general.

"So, Mom, I remember when you and I were still living in the same house, after your divorce and I returned home from college. I recall there was some conflict over the temperature in the house, especially at night. Do you remember that?"

"I really don't remember, Julie. That was so long ago."

"Well, what do you remember about going through menopause? I really need to know."

After a long pause my mom said, "Good Luck."

"Good Luck?" I responded in a heightened, irritated voice. "Good luck with what? Menopause! It's that all you're going to tell me?"

The same woman who offered me congratulations on becoming a woman, now had no words of wisdom to share about menopause or midlife in general. Feeling defeated and frustrated, I was faced with my ovaries drying up and my internal passion flame dimming at the same time on my own.

Staying open to all possibilities for myself at midlife, I gifted myself an astrology reading for my forty-seventh birthday. I had no expectations other than to tap into insight about my career. I was sensing a need to voluntarily change my working situation before an involuntary change was thrust upon me. Getting insight into midlife and menopause issues wasn't even on my radar. Could astrology really predict such things?

"So, tell me what was going on for you between the ages of 28-30?" was the first question I was asked. I thought for moment and remembered life was really good then. Actually, it was the last time in my early adult years I felt completely in own my power and happy. I had broken up with a live-in boyfriend and a year later quit my job to travel the world with only my backpack. That felt really good to remember.

"Okay! How about 35-37? What was happening then?" the astrologer asked. Ouch was all I could feel. This wasn't as pleasant to answer.

As a matter of fact, it was the darkest period of my life. I had quit a six-figure job in NYC and moved to Arizona to pursue a second chance with a past lover. What started out as an epic love story turned into a heartbreaking loss that sent me into a three-year spiraling depression. My emotions were off the chart and uncontrollable, but I didn't understand why. How could I love someone so deeply and feel so unlovable at the same time?

The phone reading continued for a total of fifty minutes with the astrologer sharing specific things about my life that people who knew me, didn't know. I was blown away, yet still unsure what this astrology stuff was all about.

The turning point was when I was presented with something to consider at the end of the session. Remember, I wanted information about my career. What she said set chills through my body.

"What I'm seeing for you is this: you can continue to experience a restless emptiness and perpetual self-loathing that no significant weight loss, bottle of expensive wine or soul-mate cosmic love would cure, or you can begin to fully embrace the unique natal map you were given and born to follow. You, Julie, are a talented speaker and coach who needs to travel the world to inspire and help others heal. In return, you experience your best self."

Today I use astrology in combination with other coaching modalities to help my clients find the validation they need to embrace what is happening in their life at the moment. Astrology has been a life-saving vehicle to help me understand the planetary cycles of my past that brought me to my present moment. Now I can embrace every stage of my life with a knowledge that the universe is always aspiring to help me learn and grow.

New to Astrology? As a 20-year Human Resources Professional followed by 10-years of operating my own company, Energetic Choices Coaching and Seminars, I felt confident in my abilities as an empowerment coach, impact speaker and retreat leader. My toolbox was full of all I needed to help women in breakdown mode learn to embrace and experience a more rich, passionate, peaceful, and deep fulfilling life… or so I thought.

Astrology, at its core, is both a language and science. It reveals cycles, archetypal patterns, and timing of certain life events. When you understand these three basics, astrology can be a wonderful self-development tool to help navigate the twist and turns of life, especially through mid-life and menopause.

Below are **three** astrology timed-events which span over an important 10–15-year period of everyone's life. I recommend for all my clients to become aware of and understand how these universal celestial events are asking each of us to grow, learn and evolve here on earth. Let us get started:

First there is Pluto Square (Ages 36-40): Ouch! When transiting Pluto was squared with my natal Pluto (a ninety-degree hard aspect) my life imploded. This transit raises power conflict on a psychological level and can bring on a physical, mental, or emotional death. During this period, I spiraled into a three-year depression and spent several years reestablishing my self-worth and personal power.

QUESTION: Was there something that died or ended or caused extreme pain? Did you let go of something or someone? Was there a change in a relationship, a career or a temporary physical or emotional pain? Did you feel like a victim or did you reclaim your inner warrior queen in the process?

Second there is Uranus Opposition (Age 40 to 42): The midlife crisis peaks here. Our worlds can be turned upside down as we look for change from a normal routine. If can feel like it is your last time to rebel. For me it was a time of great liberation, following through on my dream of speaking on big stages and coaching others to finally take bold inspired action on what really mattered to them. It became a carpe diem, seize the moment, awaking my soul to what truly mattered. I felt like I had second chance at getting my life right.

QUESTION: Did you feel a sense of wanting to break-free from all the "should"? Did you search out ways to put yourself first - ways that you never have before that might have required sudden, extreme, and revolutionary change in your life?

Third there is Neptune Square (Age 42 to 44): Neptune is known to dissolve, mystify, and ultimately transcend so it can bring on deep soul-searching. During this time, I was laid from my dream job due to the economic crisis of 2008. This allowed me to start making more honest heart-centered choices based on my passions and fulfillment over success and status. For many women, this time can also trigger perimenopausal symptoms, such as less periods. This is not the time for big life-changing decisions. Rather, this is a time to surrender to the unknown, to observe and reflect.

QUESTION? *Did you feel a sense of being lost, perhaps unmotivated or did you start to focus more on being a contribution to others versus needing to be recognized for your own success?*

Working with Julie Zolfo

Life is too short (and too long) to be anything less than fulfilled by your work, your life, your passions, and yes even your menopause journey. Up until now, you may feel like you made all the right choices for your life, but somehow your life feels wrong, off track, not so fun anymore. Can you relate?

My wish for you is… that you stay open to all possibilities, including astrology, to help you experience a complete life of joy, self-love, emotional balance, purpose, and personal fulfillment. To create your path towards fulfillment, you must first understand the internal system that is keeping you stuck in dissatisfaction, dysfunction, and delirium. That is where I come in to help as Your Life Improvement Specialist, Personal Fulfillment Mentor and Practical Astrologer.

Fulfillment is not a secret… there is a formula! Ten years ago, I created a process called *The Fulfillment Factor Formula*™ during my own personal quest to find my true north.

When it comes to fulfillment, clarity is key. And while clarifying your own unique personal path can take time, it helps to narrow down which direction you need to move in. To do that, I have created this assessment as a first step in mapping out your trajectory.

It is time to embrace your highest self. Here is the link to help you get started: **https://www.juliezolfo.com/assessment**

Once you completed the assessment, you are invited to a free DISCOVERY CALL. The intention of the free session is to have you train me on you, what you wish for in your life, and what you are willing to do differently, to create a passionate and fulfilling life.

Here is what we will cover:

▶ Why you presently feel unfilled or stuck in one or more areas of your life?

▶ What are your hopes, desires, dreams for your future?

- ▶ What results are you committed to producing?
- ▶ What do you see as a possibility for your life if you achieve your desire outcome?

The free DISCOVERY SESSION value is $150 and beyond PRICELESS when you break free of what is stopping you from having it all! Will YOU be my next be success-sister?

Blessings, Bliss and Breakthroughs,
Julie Zolfo
www.juliezolfo.com

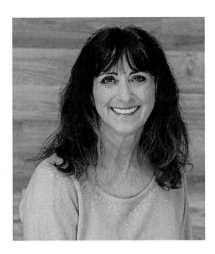

Joyce Mills Blue

"Sweet as Sugar" describes Joyce. Knowing her expertise as a financial expert, I expected to speak with someone more stoic. During our first conversation, I knew I was conversing with an exemplary woman.

Because of Joyce's personal trials turned triumphant, a burning desire burned within her to empower women in mastering their relationship with money.

Mindset and money are tightly woven and when one is off kilter, so is the other.

Joyce is a best-selling author and international speaker. It is not surprising that she has excelled. I credit her outstanding success to her merciful spirit and goodwill towards women. When Joyce is in your corner, you have a true advocate.

YOU CAN CLEAR THE FOG FROM YOUR FINANCIAL LIFE: STRATEGIES FOR FINANCIAL WELLNESS DURING MENOPAUSE

By Joyce Mills Blue

"We are not taught financial literacy in school. It takes a lot of work and time to change your thinking and to become financially literate." –Robert Kiyosaki

MONEY IS ONE OF those areas of life that has just gotten a bad rap. Many people just don't understand how money really works and have polarized it over the centuries. Money is just a tool like a screwdriver! More on that later. When adding financial stress to the stress of menopause it can be overwhelming and all-consuming, and it doesn't have to be that way at all. I want to empower you with some practical strategies and thoughts that will help you clear the fog from your finances, so you can live in peace and form an amazing, secure relationship with your finances. Are you ready?

My father was an entrepreneur and owned his own business. He always taught me that your word is your bond, and your credit score is just as important. I've been assisting others to get their finances in order for over twenty years. But my financial journey hasn't always been smooth sailing.

After starting out great and running strong with the things I had been taught, I fell in love and got married just after my twentieth birthday. I had just under $7,000.00 in the bank, and since I came from a financially secure household, I didn't know the right questions to ask before adding someone to my bank account. I was young and realized shortly into my journey that I had made a huge mistake. Money was disappearing out of the account at an alarming rate with no end in sight. Soon we were living paycheck to paycheck, and I found my new husband was more interested in partying than in paying the bills.

To make matters worse, he became very physically abusive. Six month later, all the money in the account was gone and we were in debt. This was back before direct deposit when you had to physically come home with your paycheck and deposit it into your account. I followed him out of the house one night and on to the driveway. I was trying to get some answers as to how we were going to get the bills paid and that he needed to come home with his check. I knew he didn't have time to beat me because he was on his way to work.

He got in my face, looked me right in the eyes and said, "You'll never leave me, you need me too much." Then he got in his car and drove away.

I started to cry. You see I had been a pretty fearless kid growing up with three older brothers, but this type of abuse becomes disempowering very quickly. I went inside, plopped myself on the floor and sobbed. Then I listened to the little voice inside me that said, "Hey you don't need this. You've never done anything to deserve this, and by the way you earned that money before you met him, and you can do it again!" That was the night I left.

Broke, but with a renewed flame, I moved back in with my parents that night. In two days, I had a room in a three bedroom house with coworkers and my own bank account again. I started putting the principals I had learned in my youth back to work and fine-tuned my understanding and implementation of them. In no time, I was out of debt except for my car, and paying extra on it every month to get rid of that payment as well. I started helping a few close friends by teaching them what I had done. As the years passed, I refined my system and helped even more people. In 2015, I found the neuroscience piece and realized that this was the key to why some people can fix their financial situation and thrive, and others fixed their financial situation and then end up right back where they started again or were worse in just a short time.

The Mind Game

Your mindset about this is so critical. In order for things to change, your belief and mindset needs to change. Your mindset is your beliefs, and your beliefs drive everything you do. Either you will control both your mind and your money, or both your mind and your money will control you. Did you know over 65% of the United States lives paycheck to paycheck? Even many of those that are earning in the top income brackets. If you have limiting beliefs about money stuck in your subconscious mind, you'll never get to where you want to financially. What are limiting beliefs? A *limiting belief* is something you believe to be true about yourself, about others, or about the world that limits you in some way. The challenge with *limiting beliefs* is most people don't think they have them and they can be really hard to spot. The first time I heard the phrase "***limiting belief***" I was sure I didn't have any and you may be thinking the same thing. Let me give you a quick way to find out. If you are breathing, you have them. We all have them. Here are three of the most common limiting beliefs around money:

1. Money is hard to make
2. Money is the root of all evil
3. I'm not good with money

Now that you know what limiting beliefs are, why does this matter? 80% of your success with anything is determined by your mindset. You need to focus on what you want and not the limiting belief. I have a favorite quote by Louise Hay which is, "I don't fix problems, I fix my thinking and the problems fix themselves."

Let me share two ways to transform limiting beliefs into empowering ones. One way is through affirmations. Affirmations can be very powerful but are not a quick fix. Affirmations are like brushing your teeth and need to be done multiple times a day.

Affirmations are simple and can be placed anywhere. One of Bob Proctor's favorite affirmations is "I am so happy and grateful now that..." and you can fill in the blank with whatever you want.

The second way is reframing. Reframing simply takes the negative limiting belief and reframes it into something positive. If you believe (or have been taught) that money is the root of all evil, you can simply say, "Money is a tool that I can use for my benefit."

WARNING, when you first start doing either of these, that little voice in your head is going to tell you it isn't true. Do them anyway! Thank it for its input and let it know this is your new reality and keep going.

Spending Dysfunction

Next, you need to stop spending dysfunction. Are you in the habit of paying for everything with your debit card or credit card? Women don't relate to money the way men do. Money is very linear in nature, and women are very relational. You must think of your finances as another relationship. If a friend, spouse or family member was super negative every time you were around them would you want to be around them? NO! Well money is the same way. Everything is made up of energy, including money. That's one reason it's called currency. When was the last time you made a purchase in cash? How about a cash purchase that was three or four figures? What if you did that for the next week, or better yet for the next ninety days? When you purchase things with debit or credit card, your brain does not process that transaction the same as when you physically have the money in your hands and purchase with cash. One of my clients talked about how they would see that next thing that they wanted in the store and they would get flooded with excitement, and this is exactly what happens. You get flooded with dopamine and serotonin and all these feelgood chemicals and then you purchase with a card and your brain doesn't register it as a purchase. Then the bill comes and it's like well crap, now how do I pay for this? Money has energy just like everything else. When you have money in your hands and you feel the energy of it and process that you worked for it, your conviction to get the value of whatever it is you are buying will be at much higher level and you will be more deliberate with what you purchase and if you really need it. Clients talk about how they really stopped to think if they really needed what it was they had gone to purchase when they paid with cash.

The statistic used to be if you walked into a retail establishment with a credit or debit card that you would spend on average 15% more than if you paid with cash. Now statistics show you'll spend upward of 65% more! What could you do with 15% to 65% more income at the end of the month in your personal or business budget?

Will This Really Help?

Now, none of this matter if you don't resolve to take inspired action to change your fate. That little voice inside of you is always going to try and keep you in your "comfortable patters" of doing things. Have you ever driven some place and then thought, "How did I get here?!" Your first step to changing anything is awareness. When your old ways are costing you more than they are supporting you and you become aware of this, AND accept it, change can happen. Taking action and rapid implementation is key. One client that I worked with several years ago, came to me with no idea where his money was going and just couldn't figure out why he was deep in debt. It didn't take us long to figure out his limiting beliefs and help him reframe those. He started paying with things in cash and implemented the other strategies I gave him. In one year, he was out of debt, including his car payment, and banking money like crazy to save for a new home. He was so excited and couldn't believe how different his entire life was.

I'm sure you've heard the saying knowledge is power. I'm here to tell you knowledge is not power. You can have all the knowledge in the world and if you take NO action on it, nothing changes.

Are you ready to end the struggle? I challenge you to TAKE ACTION right now by going to https://www.moremoneymethod.com and downloading my free guide on reframing and releasing limiting beliefs about money, so you can start finding those limiting beliefs that are hiding in plain sight and reach your goals.

After downloading the guide, ask yourself the following questions:

► What is one limiting belief I have about money that I want to change?

► How can I reframe that?

► What is one thing I can do today to change my financial position?

Recap

So, let's do a quick recap. First, your mindset is 80% of your success in everything you do. Also, your brain only knows what you tell it. If you're constantly telling it you'll never get a head or other negative things it will believe you! Let me give you an example. Harvard did a study where they brought in piano players and hooked them up to the brain machines. They sat them in front of the piano and had them play their favorite piece and watched what parts of their brains lit up. They then sat them in a room with no piano and had them visualize themselves playing the exact same piece on the piano with the same feeling and emotion. The exact same parts of their brains lit up!

Second, end the spending dysfunction by breaking old spending patterns and form new healthier habits when it comes to your finances. If nothing else, go get your discretionary spending money out of the bank each week and spend it in cash.

Lastly, though we have barely scratched the surface, take inspired action. Nothing with change with your situation if you don't change anything. The same thoughts and actions will NOT get you to the next level financially. Knowledge is NOT power. *Applied* knowledge is power.

Let's Connect!

Joyce Blue is a certified transformational mindset, life, business and Rapid Results coach who helps women break free of self-esteem issues and take consistent action to become financially fit, emotionally secure, and more confident so they can live the lives they love, even if they have been struggling for years. She is passionate about empowering women to master their relationship with money so all their relationships can thrive.

Her contagious energy, radiating warmth, practical strategies and thoughtful ways put her clients at ease and empower women to take inspired actions that will result in living full, happy lives with peace of mind and excitement for the future.

Joyce's entire career has been focused around helping others. After experiencing abuse and overcoming trauma herself she became committed to helping others triumph over hardships that stand in the way of them reaching their full potential. She believes that mindset, finances, life experiences and happiness are very tightly intertwined and if one is off balance it can affect your entire well-being.

She is an International and Amazon #1 bestselling author & International speaker.

She has been featured on *Let's Do Influencing, Triumph & Tiaras* and *Spiritual & Empowerment Living with Tia, Real, Raw & Relevant TV* and featured in *Focus On Fabulous Magazine, OppLoans, Fit Small Business, Newsday, Thrive Global and* more.

Joyce was born and raised in California and was the daughter of a retired Army Drill Sargent. She states: "It made for an interesting childhood, but I sure learned a lot!" She moved to the Midwest for nine years and now resides in Idaho where she works worldwide via the Internet and modern technology.

Joyce was an avid horseback rider in her younger years, and grew to love art, stain glass work and being in nature. She now enjoys genealogy, helping others and spending time with family and friends.

Joyce's Social Media Links:

Free Gift: https://www.moremoneymethod.com
Email: joyce.blue@wealthwave.com/
Facebook Business Page: https://www.facebook.com/empoweringyouLEC
Instagram: https://www.instagram.com/empoweringyouLEC

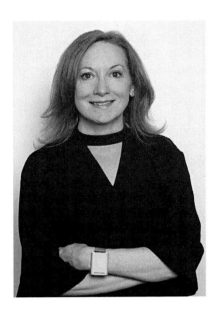

Liz Gazda

From the moment I spoke with Liz on the phone, I was compelled to align myself with her and learn from her. An intellectual woman who drives innovation for global businesses, Liz enraptures you with the ability to immediately connect on a personal level. She is an inspirer of women who transforms the ordinary into the extraordinary.

Liz is the CEO of Embr Labs, a Boston, MA based company that developed the Embr Wave, a wrist-worn wearable companion that makes temperature personal. This device improves sleep, reduces hot flashes, relieves anxiety, alters mood disturbances and cognitive impairment.

Evidence shows that thermal interventions in the body help regulate menopausal symptoms. This is a tangible solution that every woman needs.

Prior to Embr Labs, Liz was a member of several founding teams. She received her undergraduate degree in Anthropology and International relations from UC Berkeley. She also holds an International MBA and Executive coaching degree. With Liz at the helm of Embr Labs, her zealous enthusiasm has quickly brought global awareness to the Embr Wave.

WAVING GOODBYE TO HOT FLASHES

By Liz Gazda

As the CEO of Embr Labs, I've thought a great deal about how menopause should be a woman's "final frontier" - a time when she has been liberated from the cycle of menstruation, reproduction and birth control. But, as we know, menopause brings a whole new set of "challenges" - if I can use that euphemism.

Looking at the entire cycle of a woman's life has made me surmise that the best moment of a woman's life may be the age of ten. I don't mean that literally, of course. But there was something powerful about looking ahead at life from the perspective of a ten-year-old. At ten, girls have passed through the challenging stages of learning how to navigate the world. They have found themselves firmly in control and understand their environment. If you've ever seen a group of ten-year-old girls, they are confident, sassy, and ready to conquer anything that comes their way. I remember my own ten-year-old generalization. It went something like this: "I can do anything. There's no difference between opportunities for boys or girls—we both have a shot of achieving anything we want."

How different it would be. The next 40 years of my life would be marked by moments of head-shaking dismay at trying to understand why the demands of my biology put me in second place—especially in light of a woman's biological responsibility to conceive, carry, birth, nurse, nurture, and raise the next generation. As I type these words, I realize that equality is probably a low bar—perhaps hazard pay is in order.

At puberty, a girl begins 35 to 40 years of menstruation. On average, that's about 451 menstrual cycles in a lifetime, adding up to 35 years of menstrual activity, which includes planning, procuring expensive products, and laying in pain medication, as over 80% of women experience pain during their cycle with 20% experiencing pain so severe that it results in lost sleep and absenteeism from school and work. According to the website Dollars and Sense, the total financial cost that a woman will outlay to manage her period over 33 years is $17,556 at minimum. And there's more. Feminine care products are classified by the FDA as "medical devices," BUT the IRS does not acknowledge this classification, which prevents women from using pre-tax dollars in health savings accounts or flexible spending accounts to purchase the products they need.

It goes on from there. Women carry a baby to term and sacrifice careers to step away and attend to children during a child's most formative years, which we now know are critical to child development, yet the United States does not require businesses to provide paid maternity leave. For those who are able to take time off, once they return to work, they face the most basic postpartum challenges. If a woman does go back to work, the next decades of raising children can be taxing, to say the least. According to Forbes, women take ten times as much temporary leave from work as men, are eight times more likely than men to look after sick children, and 21% of women said they were paid less for doing the same work they did before they took time off to care for their children. Throw in additional factors such as caring for elderly parents and taking time to do more of the household chores, and a woman will have earned a cumulative $1,055,000 less than her male counterpart by the time she reaches retirement age.

As women age and chronic conditions set in, the healthcare system does not often succeed in supporting women. Drugs and medical devices work differently in women than in men, yet many are never adequately tested in women. According to the FDA's Office of Women's Health, women have twice the risk of developing an adverse drug reaction compared to men. In fact, until 1988, clinical trials of new drugs were conducted on predominantly male subjects, although women consumed 80% of the pharmaceuticals in the U.S. at the time.

One might surmise that this biological inequality ends once a woman reaches menopause. Menstruation is over. Reproduction is done, and there is no chance of getting pregnant. But as other biological responsibilities diminish, the decline in estrogen kicks a woman's body into a state of chaos: hot flashes, headaches, anxiety, and insomnia are just a few of the challenges that women face as they enter the final stage of their reproductive life. Some women will remain in a menopausal state for decades, with a subset experiencing up to twenty hot flashes a day. Women who experience a greater number of menopausal symptoms have been found to be significantly associated with a lower quality of life.

While the social and cultural impacts of menopause have been examined academically (though probably not enough) and anecdotally through the lived experiences of women for generations, the other impacts of menopause—particularly the economic impact—have not been researched as thoroughly. One study showed that women dealing with extensive menopause symptoms have approximately 40% higher overall costs than those who don't, stemming from both medical needs and work absence. Another study showed that women suffering from hot flashes had to pay an additional $1,649 of medical services per year, not including prescriptions or alternative medicine.

But the tide is turning: By 2025, there will be over 1.1 billion women experiencing menopause globally—12% of the entire population—and the market has taken notice. Menopause-related products and services are growing at a rapid pace and investment in new companies is quickly following. The global menopausal hot flash market is projected to reach a whopping $16B by 2027...so finally, impossible to ignore.

The time is right for innovation. Until now, the standard of care to manage menopause has been hormone replacement therapy, but the potential risk factors (including blood clots, strokes, and some cancers) have left many women searching for natural alternatives, like the Embr Wave. The Wave is a natural option that has been validated to help with hot flashes and sleep by tapping into the body's "own pharmacy". It is a beautiful wearable that allows women to access help for hot flashes "anywhere, anytime"

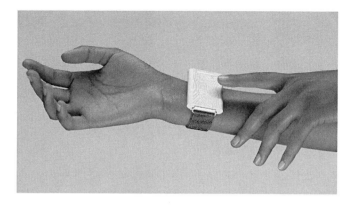

How Embr Labs became interested in solving the challenge of hot flashes

Embr Labs was founded by three materials science engineers from the Massachusetts Institute of Technology: Matt, Sam, and David. Tired of feeling constantly chilled while working in an air-conditioned lab, they got the idea for the Embr Wave, a wearable bracelet that warms or cools the sensitive skin on the inside of the wrist at the push of a button. They formed a company, took several years to build and patent their technology. Embr Labs then began producing the device and selling it directly to consumers.

Then something interesting happened.

People started writing to Embr Labs and posting reviews online describing their experiences with using the Wave. Many of them were using it to help manage health conditions that involved an inability to regulate body temperature. By far, the largest group of consumers that we heard from were women using the device to successfully manage hot flashes—not eliminating them completely, but reducing their frequency, severity, and overall bothersomeness. Others were using it to improve sleep and reduce anxiety.

With these insights, the company then partnered with Johnson & Johnson to conduct a study for women with hot flashes, and the researchers found that the Embr Wave not only improved how quickly women fell asleep and went back to sleep after waking, but the Embr Wave was shown to reduce hot flashes by up to 168%.

What we know about hot flashes

If you've ever experienced a hot flash, you know how it can interfere with your day to day activities, including sleep. And you're not alone. At menopause, 80% of women report bothersome hot flashes, with the highest frequency reported from early to late perimenopause. Several large studies have documented the negative impact of hot flashes on quality of life. No surprise, hot flashes are associated with both physical and emotional stress. In one study, participants reported that their hot flashes negatively affected their work (46.0%), social activities (44.4%), leisure activities (47.6%), sleep (82.0%), mood (68.6%), concentration (69.0%), sexual activity (40.9%), total energy level (63.3%) and overall quality of life (69.3%).

What causes hot flashes? It's certainly related to decreased levels of reproductive hormones produced as women age, and there's some evidence that our thermal comfort zone, regulated by a brain region called the hypothalamus, gets narrower as we go through menopause. When a hot flash occurs, it arises from a temporary spike in the sympathetic nervous system - which is essentially your "fight or flight" response.

Once that happens, peripheral blood vessels dilate. Blood flow increases and skin temperature in the chest, face, arms, fingers, abdomen, back, legs, and toes becomes elevated. Measureable sweating occurs in about 90% of hot flashes. And hot flashes that happen while sleeping can result in night sweats that leave women feeling chilled afterwards.

But what if you could interrupt that process, and in effect 'short-circuit' the hot flash?

Why the Embr Wave can alleviate hot flashes

Areas like the inner wrist, have highly sensitive thermoreceptors that can detect temperature changes and send signals to the brain, through a complex network that includes the somatosensory cortex, hypothalamus, anterior cingulate cortex, ventral striatum, and insular cortex. When the Embr Wave delivers cooling to the wrist, the brain then processes those temperature sensations to not only produce a feeling of cooling "whole body" relief, but the result of these cooling sensations can even "stop a hot flash in its tracks".

One of the most intriguing aspects of this process is that these regions of the brain are the same regions we use to process emotions. It's no coincidence that we use temperature metaphors to describe how we feel and respond emotionally: "hot-headed" or "warm-hearted", for example, or giving someone the "cold shoulder or a "freezing glance".

How Embr Wave works to interrupt a hot flash

Embr Wave is a bracelet that delivers either warming or cooling sensations via thermal 'waveforms'. The waveforms rise and fall in precise and consistent rhythmic patterns, and can be adjusted to deliver more or less intense thermal sensations.The amplitude and frequency of the waveforms can be individualized to provide a personalized thermal experience. A companion mobile app can be used to change or control the range of temperature settings and session duration. The bracelet uses a rechargeable battery as its power source; depending on how often sessions are initiated and the intensity of the temperature range selected, a charge can last about two days on average. And because you can start cooling or warming with the push of a button, people tell us that sometimes they use warming to offset any chill they might feel following a hot flash.

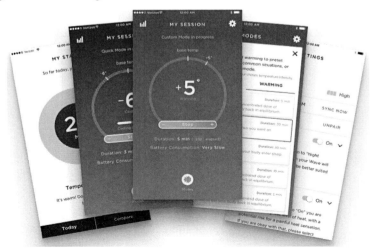

Tips for keeping your cool with Embr Wave

First time out of the box:

▶ Download the Embr Wave mobile app to get the most out of your Embr Wave. With the app you'll be able to activate various modes for longer durations, have greater temperature control, and get access to any new software updates. Follow the on-screen instructions to set up the app and pair your Embr Wave device to your phone.

▶ You can set your Embr Wave to Cooling Only so that if you accidentally press the wrong side of the light bar, your Embr Wave won't start warming. You can set this up through the app in Settings. You can also set the light bar to be dimmed or off entirely.

▶ Place Embr Wave on the inside of your wrist. The band should be snug but not uncomfortably tight. Wake up Embr Wave by pressing anywhere on the light bar until you feel it click and see the lights turn on to red and blue. Use the app to find your temperature sweet spot or start cooling or warming by pressing either side of the light bar. After activating Embr Wave, you'll quickly feel the cool or warm sensation on your wrist.

Incorporating the Wave into your daily routine:

▶ Embr Wave warms or cools in waves. Gently focus your attention on the waves of temperature. Let your body relax. Take slow, easy breaths and focus on the sensations you're experiencing.

▶ **Essential Mode** is the default mode on your Embr Wave. Sessions in Essential Mode last for ten minutes. Use Essential Mode throughout the day reactively when you feel a hot flash coming on and proactively even when you are not experiencing them.

▶ **Quick Mode** is a short, 3-5 minute session on Embr Wave. In this mode, the waves are fairly quick and intense. Some people use Quick Mode cooling first thing in the morning to help establish a daily routine. Or use it after a warm shower, blow drying your hair, or any activity that could trigger a hot flash.

Fall Asleep Mode:
► Before going to bed at night, you can switch cooling or warming functionality to Fall Asleep Mode. In this mode, the sessions last for 35 minutes and the waves are timed to follow the rhythm of relaxed breathing.. And, the light bar is muted to help keep your room dark.

All Night Mode
► All night mode was especially designed for gentle all night cooling to keep you comfortable and provide a defence against those irritating night-time hot flashes!

Bio

Elizabeth Gazda is the CEO of Embr Labs, a Boston-based wearables company that developed the Embr Wave – a wrist-worn, personal thermostat that improves sleep, relieves anxiety and helps with hot flashes.

Prior to Embr Labs, Liz was a member of several founding teams including Doni, a fintech company, and Noteflight, a music technology company and has also worked at a number of Boston's fastest growing companies, including m-Qube (acq. Verisign) and unicorn Art Technology Group (acq. Oracle). Liz began her career with Philips Consumer Electronics in the Netherlands, where she was responsible for driving innovation in several business divisions across multiple countries.

Elizabeth received her undergraduate degree in Anthropology and International relations from UC Berkeley where she was also a member of the Women's Varsity Soccer team. She also holds an International MBA from Nijenrode University in the Netherlands and an Executive Coaching degree from William James College.

Elizabeth serves as a board member and advisor to several Boston-based startups in IoT, hardware and software.

Website: https://embrlabs.com
Instagram: https://www.instagram.com/embrlabs/
Facebook: https://www.facebook.com/embrlabs/

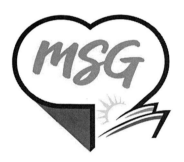

The best part about life is that EVERY MORNING you have the opportunity to become a happier version of yourself.

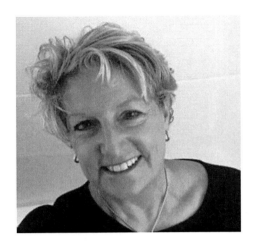

Amy Buckalter

When you are in Amy's space, you feel like you've entered into a fantasy land. Amy is an ingenious inventor who tells a story like no one I know. She takes you into her world of imagination without you even knowing you've entered. When you're there, you know you are in the presence of greatness.

Amy possesses a discerning vision that ultimately birthed her invention. Through unrelenting perseverance, she brought her invention to market and is changing lives globally.

When I first met Amy in her lab, I was captivated by her ability to execute with unfeigned good humor, keeping everyone engaged and involved, which are traits of a true champion.

Amy is a trusting, brilliant, genuine, energetic, and loyal friend. She uses her prowess to overachieve so others can benefit. What a gift.

PULSE: LUXURIOUSLY TRANSFORMING YOUR PERSONAL LUBRICANT EXPERIENCE

By Amy Buckalter

I F THERE'S A LIFE event that puts you on notice, makes you go hmmmmm, and compels you to whisper "OMG" all at the same time…it's midlife and the onset of menopause. As many women, I became aware that something was drastically changing with my body when my "internal faucets" began to turn off, vaginal dryness ensued, and with it, discomfort and pain during sex. *Sigh…*

My gynecologist explained that this was a sign of perimenopause and from now on, as I moved into full blown menopause and beyond, this would be my "new normal". With this new and disheartening information, so began my use of personal lubricants; the #1 non-hormonal physician recommended solution for relieving pain from vaginal dryness. Unlike many younger women today who use lubricants (not because they need it, but because it just makes intimacy better and more comfortable), my generation was introduced to lube because it was necessary to soothe our discomfort. I tried so many different options… including those that were recommended by doctors and experts alike. I found every one of them truly inconvenient, messy, and uncomfortably cold (talk about a mood killer!). I wrapped bottles and tubes in heating pads or submerged them in warm water baths – anything to reduce the disruptive chill. They were lacking and annoying in many other ways as well — some left me more dry than moisturized, some irritated my most sensitive tissues, most were sticky and gross, and were full of questionable ingredients (who wants petrochemicals, parabens, and glycerin in our most sensitive of body parts)? I had to ask myself, "Really, is this it…is this as good as it gets?" I was increasingly frustrated and turned off by the outdated clinical experience of a cold, sticky, and unhygienic tube or bottle, as well as lubricant products that included dangerously unhealthy ingredients. Why after a 100 hundred years of personal lubricants being available on the market, with more than 65% of all women using lubricants to relieve pain, thirty-one million women experiencing menopause each year, and 58% of post-menopausal women experiencing vaginal dryness, had there been no significant improvement to this unpleasant and dated experience? With that question in mind, I set out to better understand if other women were equally dissatisfied with this archaic, but much needed, lubricant solution and the user experience. I hired a PhD researcher to work with me to survey 300-400 women to explore their unmet needs with lubricant use… was it similar to mine or was I the only one with this jaded opinion about lube? Not only did I discover similarity in perspectives, but the information gathered was extremely educational; I learned that almost every respondent had something negative to say in describing their experiences: "awkward", "embarrassing", "icky", "gross", "inconvenient", "uncomfortably cold", "disruptive to the moment", "messy", "hard to control dispensing the amount desired", "unhealthy ingredients", and the list goes on. That was the defining moment for me…the moment when I decided it was time to transform and modernize the personal lubricant solution because every woman deserves a better experience than what she has had to accept for decades. Every woman deserves to have comfortable intimacy, a desirable and welcoming solution rather than a clinically cold or embarrassing remedy, and a seamless connection with her partner rather than awkward and interrupted moments. Her improved quality of life means not having to settle or compromise her sexual health needs, or her emotional and physical well-being, because of being confronted by the changes of her body during this life stage and then having to choose between poorly developed or unhealthy available options or, nothing at all. I was compelled to create a modern and elegant solution for all of us. In the late Spring of 2013, I set off on my journey to do just that... During my initial research previously mentioned, whereby I wanted to validate that yes, women are not satisfied with their personal lubricant experience, the research identified the following issues. It also allowed us to comprehend what we needed to build so to not only solve the issues, but to make the entire experience inviting, convenient, comfortable, and healthy.

Over the next five years, we formed a team of highly committed and passionate Strategic Advisors, consultants, board directors, business partners, and a few full-time employees – all of whom worked tirelessly to ideate, design, engineer, test, manufacture, and market an innovation that would not only meet, but exceed, the expectations of our vision. Four of our advisors, who are also investors in the business, were members of the original Sonicare and Clarisonic product development teams; personal care companies introducing first to market inventions that went on to be successfully acquired and then further expanded (Sonicare by Philips and Clarisonic by L'Oréal). These advisors had tribal knowledge of the development process of personal care and medical devices that would be invaluable for us as we too were inventing something complex, and would also require clearances by the FDA as well as other manufacturing certifications. These advisors were also instrumental in guiding our development of a strong IP (intellectual property) strategy that now consists of a large portfolio of global patents and trademarks, important for protecting our invention from "copycats" and supporting our future global growth. This brilliant innovation would of course also require a large amount of capital to fund each of the many stages involved from concepting the idea to actual commercialization - market introduction and promotion. I will always be incredibly grateful for our generous investors, for without their support of our vision, this invention and business venture would not have been possible. Over the course of five years, I have been fortunate to raise a significant level of funds to support the development of the invention and business operations to take us to this point on our growth trajectory; approximately ten million dollars from individual Angel investors, all highly enthusiastic about Pulse's potential to transform, reinvent, and improve the quality of life for so many. 65% of our investors are women, which makes the funds raised even more unique and special, since generally speaking women account for only 22% of all Angel investments.

Say hello to Pulse...like a Nespresso or Keurig for the bedroom.

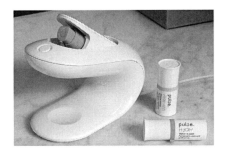 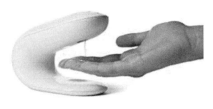

Pulse and Pulse Pods is the world's first device and consumable delivery platform designed to significantly transform consumer experience with creams, oils, lotions, gels, and any substance in a liquid consistency. Pulse is a stylish modern designed device that conveniently andautomatically, dispenses lubricant formulations in comfortably warm, clearn, and precise doses. Pulse eliminates that unwanted mess (from overpours and limited portion control), the contamination and bacteria that accompany sticky surface residues, and the crusty build-up around nozzles or rims, and removes those unpleasant chilly temperatures that make relaxation of sensitive vaginal tissue way more challenging and are simply uncomfortable. No more fumbling around in your night table drawer trying to find that sticky bottle of lub; Pulse is easily accessible and ready to serve your needs when you desire. These are all issues found with lubricants when dispensed from traditional bottles and tubes.

Pulse, Where Nespresso functionality meets Apple design for Personal Care

The Pulse Platform

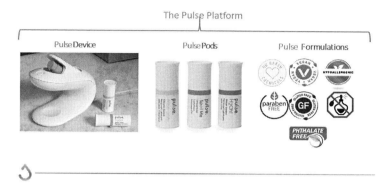

Pulse Device   Pulse Pods   Pulse Formulations

Pulse Pods are small chic containers that look like cosmetics or lipsticks and they are filled with Pulse's proprietary healthy and luxurious FDA-cleared personal lubricants. Once the Pod is inserted into the Pulse device, they are safely warmed and hygienically dispensed into one's hand upon motion activated request. No mess, no inconvenience, and no uncomfortable cold. Instead, a convenient, welcoming, clean and comfortable experience. There's truly nothing like it. And to align our Pulse Pods with environmental sensitivity, our Pulse Pods are recyclable.

Pulse Pods... chic, convenient, and healthy

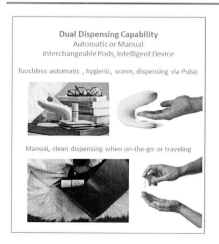

Dual Dispensing Capability
Automatic or Manual
Interchangeable Pods, Intelligent Device

Touchless automatic , hygienic, warm, dispensing via Pulse

Manual, clean dispensing when on-the-go or traveling

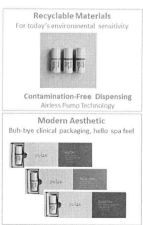

Recyclable Materials
For today's environmental sensitivity

Contamination-Free Dispensing
Airless Pump Technology

Modern Aesthetic
Buh-bye clinical packaging, hello spa feel

When we were developing Pulse and Pulse Pods, we first focused on the dispensing technology itself; that which that would make the experience comfortably warm, clean and hygienic, mess-free, and extremely convenient. What we didn't know right from the beginning, was the type of lubricant that we would we be offering in our lubricant Pods. Would we allow any company to create Pulse Pods of their lubricants and use our Pulse device as their dispensing platform? Or would we perhaps private label a lubricant company's brand that we believed was a superior lubricant in the market? As we began to consider options, we determined that there was nothing exceptional enough in the market offerings to pair with our exceptional device. Although there were healthier, more natural and organic lubricant options arriving in the market, they suffered from icky-stickiness and irritating added frangrances. After much consideration, we decided that we would take the more difficult road of developing and FDA clearing our own proprietary formulations. Yes, it would be lengthy, and yes it would be expensive... but of high priority was creating a truly extraordinary, healthy, and luxurious product; unmatched by anything available on the market. One of our amazing talented advisors, who is a very experienced naturopathic physician and is a specialist in female health, began working with us and our chemists to create two best in market product options; a premium silicone-based lubricant and a natural water-based lubricant.

Pulse Formulations

Sets new superior benchmark

o Healthy Ingredients, No Harmful Chemicals
o Natural Feel, Not Sticky
o Unscented & Hypoallergenic
o Hydrating and Soothing
o Contamination - free airless pump technology
o Recyclable Packaging
o Dispensed manually, or, automatically via Pulse
o All required FDA approvals are issued

Aloe-ahh
Silicone-Based
With
Aloe + Vitamin E

H2Oh!
Natural Water-Based
With
Pure Chia Extract

Spoil Me
A Blend
of Six
Natural Oils

Pulse's silicone-based product would use only a medical grade silicone, rich and exceptional in quality and include ingredients with soothing healing properties. Our "Aloe-ahh" was developed to be just that; soothing, and includes aloe and vitamin E known for its healing characteristics. Our natural water-based formulation, H2Oh!, took over 137 iterations to ensure that it was not only meeting the objective of superior hydration, but also luxurious in its feel. Most water-based formulations tend to be sticky or actually dehydrating as they can either include chemicals that dry the tissues, or perhaps include too much aloe or other ingredients not in proper ratio. We abandoned many of the usual ingredients and set out to find something unique, natural, and exceptionally hydrating that would also provide silkiness and not stickiness; so, the feel would mimic one's own natural body lubrication. Our advisor and naturopathic physician identified the perfect magical ingredient … pure chia extract from organic chia seeds. It's a total WOW! We are now the only brand in the world, that we know of, that is using this remarkable ingredient with properties that offer the benefits of both superior hydration and surpurb slip. In terms of hydration, the World Health Organization (WHO) has deemed the optimal level of osmolality to be 380. Osmolality in lay person's terms measures hydration. The higher the number, the worse and more dehydrating to the vaginal tissues, the lower the number, the better and more hydrating. The WHO states between 380 and 1200 is acceptable. Any higher osmolality is dehydrating and with friction can cause tears in the tissue and allow for unwanted STDs or STIs if unprotected. The lower the number, even better! Pulse's H2Oh! natural water-based formula measures better than optimally hydrating at 301. Isn't hydration and comfort the purpose of using lubricant?!

Our Pulse innovation debuted to the market in 2017 and has been adding raving fans by the day. Since launching, 95% of the customer and physician reviews on our website are 5-star and we have had less than 1% product returns. We have also been quite impressed to see that 40% of our buyers are men, demonstrating their desire to improve the quality of comfortable intimacy within their relationships, and recognizing that when their female partner is more comfortable, sexual intimacy is simply "better". During our development progress, our Pulse innovation has evolved into a solution with significant implications and tremendous potential. Sexual wellness is our first application because relieving discomfort from vaginal dryness during menopause was a vital objective and my inspiration for the invention; I was compelled to create a modern, convenient, and healthy solution. What we have come to realize over time, is that many personal care, healthcare, and even beauty products in liquid form would benefit from being dispensed in a convenient, clean-hygienic, comfortably warm (or in the future, also cooled) manner, and in precise dosage. Future applications we envision as benefiting from our Pulse platform will be in the categories of baby care, skincare, and facial care amongst others. All of us on the Pulse team imagine a world where Pulse remarkably transforms and improves the consumer experience with endless personal care applications in the same way that Nespresso and Keurig transformed and improved their coffee experience. A Pulse in every room and an abundance Pulse Pod options for every Pulse.

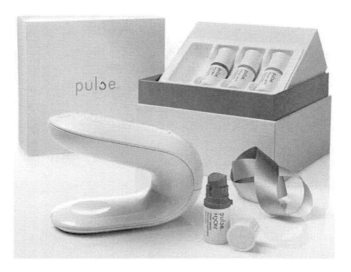

Looking back at where we began, and now looking forward with a line of sight on our exciting future possibilities, I have menopause to thank for inspiring us to design this brilliant transformative innovation. Here's to each of us embracing our best quality of life so we can truly thrive in every stage and phase of our existence. Pulse, for the comfort we all deserve.

Bio

Amy Buckalter
Founder and CEO

Amy Buckalter is the founder and CEO of Pulse; the world's first device and consumable platform developed to modernize and significantly improve consumers' experience with their personal care, healthcare, and beauty formulations; (lotions, oils, gels, creams, and lubricants). Pulse; think stylish Apple design meets the functional convenience and technical elegance of Keurig and Nespresso.

Pulse and Pulse Pods solve all the unpleasant and annoying issues inherent to using tubes and bottles of personal care formulations; messy overpours, bacterial contamination, handling those icky-sticky surface residues, and the fumbling around with opening and closing of caps and twist off tops. Of primary benefit, Pulse comfortably warms the formulations to increase effectiveness and eliminate those unwelcomed cold temperatures. Pulse has patented technologies for touchless motion activated dispensing, closed delivery for a clean-hygienic dispensing experience, and safe inductive warming. Additionally, the company has developed its own proprietary FDA approved healthy and luxurious formulations that have exceeded customers' expectations and raised the quality bar for competitors in their categories.

An inspiring team leader, business strategist, and operational game changer, Amy is passionate about being a market disruptor in whichever space she focuses. She has built an outstanding record of revenue achievement and value creation across the entire corporate spectrum. Her expertise includes a series of progressive leadership roles within publicly-held, privately-owned, and private equity-funded B2C organizations, as well as strategic turnaround engagements and interim executive assignments. Her 35-year career includes a variety of executive leadership roles with brand icons Nike, K2, Rollerblade, Burton, and Ellesse where she was the catalyst to accelerate growth, execute high performance turn-around results for future acquisitions, or take the business from a market challenger to a market leader position. Amy also built and led her own growth strategy consultancy, Pivot Partners LLC, helping companies and organizations "pivot" to new levels of revenue and profit.

During Amy's career, she has participated on several for-profit and non-profit Boards of Directors, including a private equity owned company resulting in a successful exit. Amy continues to be committed to mentoring MBA students and inspiring early stage entrepreneurs who are fueled by a dream to create something better and different.

Amy holds a BA double major in Economics and Sociology from Hamilton College, and has completed Executive Study in Finance from the Wharton School at the University of Pennsylvania. Amy and the Pulse organization are located in Seattle, Washington.

Pulse Website: https://lovemypulse.com/
Facebook: https://www.facebook.com/lovemypulseforever/
Instagram: https://www.instagram.com/lovemypulse/
Founder, Amy Buckalter's LinkedIn: https://www.linkedin.com/in/abuckalter/

There's going to be very painful moments in your life that will change your entire world in a matter of minutes. These moments will change YOU. Let them make you stronger, wiser and kinder. Don't become someone that you're not. Cry. Scream if you have to. Then, straighten out your crown and press on.

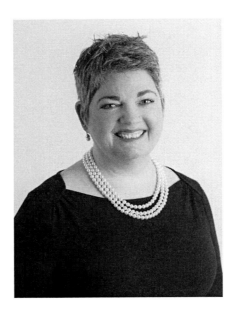

Dr. Martha Menard

If you marry humility with genius, you have met Martha. A former massage therapist who earned her PhD in quantitative and qualitative research, Martha and her husband reside in Bellingham, WA where she works as the founder and CEO of Nautilus Financial. She brings her background in psychology, education and financial wellness to help women gain greater financial flexibility and build long term wealth and financial security.

As a post menopausal woman, Martha is passionate about her work. Martha understands from first hand experience, the symptoms of menopause and how the anxiety from hormonal changes acclaim financial stress.

Martha is a refined, determined, poised, amiable woman with a vision for change. Menopause is a global epidemic that is not a discriminator of age. Martha's passion allows her to coach women of all ages. Financial wellness is preeminent to personal peace.

HOW I WENT FROM BEING CLUELESS ABOUT MONEY TO FINANCIAL BADASSERY

By Dr. Martha Menard

W HILE I ORIGINALLY TRAINED TO be a behavioral research scientist, I'm currently working as a personal finance writer, educator, and coach. I've spent the past five years working in the financial services industry. I've gone from having a negative net worth to being able to live off my investments once I'm ready to retire in a few years. But I have a confession to make.

I haven't always had a positive relationship with money. In fact, how I've learned about personal finance is the same way most people do — through making mistakes.

My Story

I grew up in a barely middle-class family that struggled with money, and the messages I absorbed were: money is hard — hard to get and hard to hold on to — and there will never be enough.

I was an emancipated minor who worked part-time all through high school and paid my way through college and grad school. I eventually earned a doctorate and built a successful business that I loved. I bought a house and was making more than decent money. Yet, between credit cards, student loans, and a home equity loan, I had almost $100,000 in debt.

In spite of having all the outward symbols of success, I felt an underlying anxiety about money most of the time. I had a little cushion in savings, but like almost 80% of Americans, I was really living paycheck-to-paycheck. And like another 45% of Americans, I had nothing saved for retirement. Zero. Zip. Nada.

The pivotal moment? When I realized that if I didn't do something, I was going to be working 40+ hours a week until I died. And that doing something to change my situation was possible. The latter was the most important— mindset is key.

I knew it was up to me, so I started learning about personal finance by reading everything I could. I learned a great deal about the dos and don'ts of managing money. But the one book that opened my eyes was *Your Money or Your Life* by Joe Dominguez and Vicki Robin. It completely transformed how I thought and felt about money, and I often recommend it to my clients.

The gist of the book is that those of us who work for a living are trading our time and our life energy for money. So when we spend money, we are really spending our life energy. And of course time is something you can only spend once.

That's a profound concept, and it really changed how I spent money going forward. The question I started asking was "Is this thing worth the time and life-energy it is really costing me?"

What was most transformative

Reading this book made me think about my then-current relationship with money, the money scripts I inherited from my family, and what I wanted my future relationship to look like. It gave me hope that it was possible to have a different relationship with money. That I could be 'good' with money. But it wasn't easy, and it didn't happen overnight.

The first time I looked at my total assets (how much money I had) and compared that amount to my total liabilities (how much money I owed), I sat down and cried. I felt completely overwhelmed. At the same time, I realized that if I were going to change my situation, I needed to make a plan.

My immediate goal was to start paying down the credit card debt I had. And as I did that, I started to change my beliefs about money.

I became more intentional about spending it, more focused on getting out of debt, and realized that to build real wealth over the long term, I need to learn how to invest.

What happened next

Once I started implementing my plan, a funny thing happened. Even though I knew it was going to take time to get to where I wanted to be financially, I noticed that I was a lot less stressed about money. I still had occasional moments or situations when I worried about a specific money issue, but the constant, low-level anxiety about money was gone. I felt lighter.

It wasn't a quick process. Tracking my progress every month and celebrating milestones helped. Once I had some emergency savings and had made a dent in paying off all my credit card debt, I started an investment account with just $50 at an online brokerage. I committed to automatically depositing another $50 a month, all the while learning about investing. I made a lot of mistakes and learned from them, and continued to read everything I could. Slowly, my dividend income increased every quarter, and then every year.

Then another funny thing happened. Friends started asking me for advice about money. Maybe it was because I had become more comfortable talking honestly about money and my own path. I wanted to help — if I could help others avoid making some of the mistakes that I had, that would be a good thing.

I started thinking about becoming a financial coach. I studied with several people, worked for a financial wellness tech startup, and even made money writing about personal finance and investing as a freelancer. I still hang out (virtually) with a group of financial coaches.

Why I'm writing this chapter

As I've gained experience, I've realized that a lot of personal finance advice is designed for an ever-shrinking group: people who have the kind of job that provides a steady salary and paid benefits. An increasing number of people simply don't. Since the 1970s, wages have stagnated while costs for housing, education, and healthcare have spiraled upward.

Many Americans live in a state of financial precarity with irregular hours, increasing costs just for basic needs, and shrinking paychecks that make it hard to save anything. The 'pull yourself up by your bootstraps and just stop buying lattes' advice doesn't work for people who don't even have boots.

We are living in an age of massive, systemic inequality. Yet a lot of traditional financial advice assumes that every individual has complete control over their financial situation and that if someone is struggling, then it must be all their own fault. Most of us have some degree of money shame, and think that we should be somehow 'be better' with money than we are.

One of the few good things that may come out of the current pandemic and associated financial meltdown we are currently experiencing could be the realization that as a nation, our government needs to do more to help its people in terms of promoting economic equality for everyone. I alternate between being hopeful and then feeling like I'm not going to hold my breath waiting for that to happen.

At the same time, until we have created a level playing field for everyone, there are a few things that the average person can do on an individual level. In this uncertain world and time of rapid change, there's a huge need for all of us to start building financial resilience and flexibility. Having more than one income source is always a good idea, but I think that now it's essential.

It's also essential to start saving for retirement, if you haven't already. Almost half of all women who receive Social Security depend on it for 90% of their income in retirement. While the average benefit is now roughly $1500 a month, that figure doesn't take into account women's typically lower lifetime earnings. Thanks to the gender pay gap, and taking time out of the workforce to provide unpaid caregiving, the average monthly Social Security benefit for women is only $1,196. That's below poverty level!

Your best financial year ever could start today

The first step in improving your financial situation is believing that change is really possible. Having a concrete plan that you can live with is the key. Here are some steps, month by month, that almost anyone can take. Try them all or just pick a few.

Months 1-2: Look at where you are, think about where you want to be, run the numbers to figure out how to get there

The first step on your journey to financial wellness is realizing where you're starting from. It's incredibly helpful to see all of your spending and savings in one place, so that you have a clear picture of all your assets, liabilities, and cash flow—how much cash you have coming in and going out every month.

If you are already using an app like Mint or Quicken, or even an Excel spreadsheet, great. If not, there are a ton of personal finance applications out there—check out the reviews on https://investorjunkie. com/personal-finance/ or https://thewirecutter.com/money/ to find one that sounds appealing to you. My favorite free personal finance app is Personal Capital (www.personalcapital.com). It's a comprehensive tool that you won't outgrow. Did I mention that it's free?

Once you know where you stand financially, it's time to think about what your goals are. Is owning a home important to you? Helping children with their educational expenses? Are there other big ticket items you want to work towards, like starting your own business? Where would you like to be financially in 5 years, 10 years, or when you're ready to stop working full-time? Knowing your financial 'why' makes it easier to say 'no' to spending temptations when you can see your 'yes'.

Once you're clear on your goals, you can create a plan that will let you get there from where you are now. Unless you're the kind of person who likes to keep a detailed budget, keep it simple: 50% of your take home goes to fixed expenses like rent and car payments, 20% to discretionary expenses like food, clothing, and entertainment, and 30% to saving toward your goals and paying off debt.

Month 3: Build or add to your emergency fund

Cars break down, pets get sick...stuff always happens. Did you know that almost 50% of Americans can't handle a $400 emergency without going into debt? Don't be one of them.

If you don't already have an emergency fund, this is the time to start one. If you are getting a tax refund this year, take half of it and use it to start your 'expect the unexpected' fund.

And especially if you are self-employed, you need a cushion for those slow weeks or months. Aim for an amount that will cover 6 months of your fixed expenses. If you have a steady paycheck and a job that's unlikely to end suddenly, you can probably get by with 3 months' worth. Adding even $20-$50 a month will build your fund up faster than you think. Keep it in a separate savings account. If you only do one thing on this list, do this one.

Month 4: Start paying down credit card debt

By now, if you're using an app to track your finances, you've got a pretty good idea of where your money is going. This is the month to start paying down any outstanding credit card debt. Start with the one that has the highest interest rate. Put the most you can afford towards that one and pay the minimum on the rest. Once you get rid of the highest interest debt, move on to the next one, and repeat the same process.

Another option that works is to start with the card that has smallest amount of debt. Some people prefer this approach because it's more motivating to see the rapid progress you can make. Again, once you've paid off that card, go on to the next.

If the idea of being debt-free is appealing, there are ways you can get there faster. Usually there's a limit on how much you can save by cutting back your spending, but there's no limit on how much you can earn. Take on some extra clients, get a temporary part-time job or start a side hustle. Put the extra money towards paying down debt more quickly or building up your emergency fund.

Month 5: Clean house and automate your finances

By now, you're making real progress at building up your savings and paying down debt. This is a good time to take stock of your overall situation. Are you spending money on what's meaningful to you? Review your subscriptions and get rid of any that you don't really use or enjoy. Ever gotten hit with a big late fee? Prevent that from happening by setting up automatic bill payments with your bank. And if your bank charges high fees to maintain your accounts, consider moving them—check out Bankrate.com. Credit unions usually offer the same services without the fees that big banks typically charge.

Month 6: Create a plan for your holiday spending

It's not too early to start thinking about your holiday spending plan. Between gifts and/or travel, it's common for people to go into debt. One study found that 56% of holiday shoppers rack up credit card debt, and many of them planned to go into debt again the following year—including people who are still paying off previous years' bills.

Decide how much you're willing to spend, and start saving now. You can also decide how you want to handle the holidays—like setting a limit on presents, just buying gifts for the kids, or taking a 'secret Santa' approach instead of buying presents for everyone. You'll save money and have less clutter. And when you do buy, take advantage of discount codes and coupons.

Month 7: Take a look at your insurance

The purpose of insurance is to reduce your financial risk. Lots of people have policies that aren't a good fit—they're either over-insured or under-insured. For example, you could be paying for more auto insurance than you really need, like collision coverage for a car that's older and worth less currently compared to when you bought it.

For anyone who is working to earn a living, disability insurance is especially important—you need to protect your income in case you can't work for some period of time, and many employers offer low cost plans through your employee benefit package.

If you're young and relatively healthy, consider a high deductible health insurance plan with a Health Savings Account. Invest the money in a low cost index fund that tracks the S&P 500, and you can use that to cover future medical expenses.

Month 8: Be mindful about where and what you spend on food
It's easy to spend money eating out—lunch with a friend, a drink after work, picking up dinner on the way home because it's late and you've had a long day. But eating out often can add up to a bigger chunk of your budget than you might like. Plus, you're more likely to let what's already in the fridge go bad. According to one study, the average American family spends over $3,000 annually on food away from home, and throws away $1,000 to $2,000 in wasted food every year.

If you kept half your eating-out spending and didn't waste as much of your grocery budget, you could invest about $3,000 annually. And if you started at age 35 and invested that amount in an Roth IRA with, say, a conservative average of 7% returns, that amount would turn into roughly $283,000 by age 65.

So make a weekly meal plan. Schedule going out for meals and decide in advance which you'll eat at home, and only buy the groceries you need. Take leftovers for lunch the next day so they don't go to waste. Plan to dine out when it's less expensive, or check Groupon for local deals. Breakfast is always my favorite.

Month 9: Turn unwanted items into cash
Take the stuff you don't use, don't need, or don't wear and sell it. Have a garage sale with neighbors, take it to a consignment shop, or sell it on eBay or Facebook Marketplace. Take the money and set it aside for month10, when you're going to celebrate your success. And enjoy your newly de-cluttered space.

Month 10: Reward yourself
You've made a lot of progress!

Use this month to review your goals, whether you're on track to meeting them, and what you need to do next. Take the money you just made from selling your unwanted stuff and do something personally meaningful with it—make a memory with friends or family, donate a sum to a favorite charity, or take a road trip. Research shows that spending money on experiences, rather than stuff, actually makes us happier. So does spending money on others.

By making even a few of these changes and building on your successes each month, you'll be less stressed about money and in better shape financially in less than a year.You'll be in a position to start making progress toward longer term financial goals. Take time to savor your wins and celebrate all that you've accomplished. Think of what you can do next!

Consider working with a financial coach

It really is possible to change your financial situation by making changes to your financial behaviors. Start with just one small step.

Some people are highly motivated and can make changes like the ones described on their own. But most of us, while we know what we should do, find that actually getting around to doing it is more challenging. That's one of the reasons I decided to go into coaching as a profession—behavior change isn't easy.

As a coach, I can only work with one person or business at a time. That's why I've decided to start offering group coaching. You can find out more by visiting my website at marthamenard.com. My goal with group coaching is to offer evidence-based information, banish money shame, and empower women to do what they can improve their financial situation, all at an affordable cost. I also offer a free phone consultation to see if coaching is a good fit for you at this point in your life.

I see money as a tool that provides us more choices for living a meaningful and generous life. It all starts with your mindset and your emotions. Understanding our beliefs and feelings about money is the key to making lasting changes in our financial behaviors and reaching our goals.

Nautilusfinancialcoaching.com

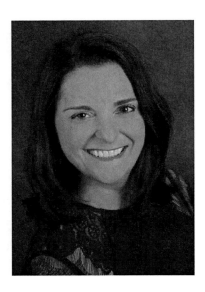

Tina McDermott

As soon as you interact with Tina, you're convinced that she's been your lifelong friend even though you never spoke before. This forthwith bond is without doubt, a result of Tina's personal inspiration of love and wellness to all. Losing her sister at the age of 23 to cancer was a wake up call for Tina to learn more about how to take better care of herself and advocate for others.

A life long sufferer of Lyme disease had Tina believing that she was menopausal at 37. When she embraced a healthy lifestyle, she was symptom free within 5 years. Now that she is 52 and actually going through menopause, Tina is cruising through this transition with grace and ease.

Tina works out of her studio in Maryland, coaching individual clients, leading small groups and teaching nutrition and cooking classes to corporations as a keynote speaker. Her programs include "Finally Thin Forever", a digital weight release course that compliments her recipe books and fitness routines.

Tina is an expert weight release coach and is passionate about helping women release unwanted weight naturally and KEEPING IT OFF FOREVER.

LEARNING TO LOVE MY BODY

by Tina McDermott

This chapter is for you if…

A. You want to lose weight, but don't know where to start

B. You've made some progress, but you're not quite as far along as you want to be. You are frustrated, wondering if you're ever going to lose weight and keep it off. You desire rapid weight loss and want to keep it off forever without yo-yo dieting

C. Your weight loss is on fire, and you're looking for some hacks to get there even faster

Which one are you?

I'm here to share some good news… If you haven't found success, IT'S NOT YOUR FAULT! You have tried all those FAD DIETS out there, and followed the rules precisely. Here's the problem… you may have some emotional baggage that needs to be permanently checked-in, and you don't have the support you need to be successful!

All that ends today. Today is the day you are going to discover how you can lose weight without starving yourself. You'll learn how you can crush cravings without depriving yourself of yummy foods. You'll explore ways to keep the weight off forever… without yo-yo dieting.

So you may be thinking, why should you listen to me? An expert would be someone who's been working with people for more than five years… helping them to attain permanent weight loss. By that definition, I'm an expert. I've actually been providing coaching and counseling for over twenty years. I'm using my certifications, and my extensive learning to help folks who are struggling and going through a painful weight loss experience.

In 2006, I started developing my *Finally Thin Forever* program. I've written all of my many lectures, programs, workbooks, and recipe books by myself. These programs have been written and tested hundreds of times with my one-on-one clients, and in small coaching groups over the years. *Finally Thin Forever* is my love, my passion, my baby. Now I'm ready to share it with you!

My Story… The Struggle is Real!

I was the third female child in an Italian family. In traditional Italian families, a boy is like royalty. He will carry on the family name. My dad so badly wanted a boy. And then… Surprise! "It's a girl!"

All joking aside, as I grew older, I could feel my Dad's disappointment. At the same time, I felt neglected by my Mom because she was emotionally unavailable. She had a host of emotional and physical challenges, which she carries with her to this day. They have only become magnified over the years.

So, the only way for me to get the love and attention I craved was to refuse food. Italian mothers take notice, reacting strongly and swiftly when kids don't eat. Unfortunately, it wasn't long before this behavior turned into **anorexia**. I became so skinny that my Nonna (Italian for Grandmom) would tell me the wind was going to blow me away. I used my refusal to eat as a form of control over my crazy Italian parents and my chaotic life. And then, for some reason, everything changed. When I was twelve years old and went to Italy with my Nonna for the summer, I fell in love with food. I was no longer anorexic… yeah!

I gained twenty pounds that summer and for the first time, I actually felt and looked healthy… with the exception of the stretch marks. But **my sisters would tease me** all the time, saying that I was fat. Please understand, I love my sisters and they did their best. However, this teasing **led to emotional eating and an obsession with exercise and losing weight**. Like so many people before me, I discovered I had an **emotional attachment to food**. Trying to regain control, I started yo-yo dieting and became an exercise fanatic for years. This caused my metabolism to become unstable.

Stressing over my exercise obsession, and my weight, caused me to have belly issues that were debilitating. Every day I was suffering from bad gas pains and bloating in my stomach, along with severe constipation.

It was so embarrassing as the gas would escape at very inconvenient times. My family even called me "Putza" which means **stinky** in Italian. The name-calling led to even **more emotional issues**.

My older sister, Anna, was diagnosed with cancer at the age of 24. Unfortunately, she lost her battle with cancer, and it took her life at the age of 48. I thought that I would probably be next because I was always sick.

Her journey was a wakeup call for me to learn more about how to take better care of myself. I never wanted to suffer as she did.

I also suffered from chronic Lyme disease and thought I was going through menopause at the age of 37. It took five years for me to get to a point when I was symptom-free. I managed this naturally through food, fitness, and the support of my loving husband of 18 years. Now that I am 53, and going through perimenopause, I have learned to embrace the transition and go through it with grace and ease.

Over the years, I began eating better and learned everything there was to know about natural health that I could. I was passionate and taught anyone who would listen. It was then that I realized it was my mission to teach wellness.

I also discovered methods to release my emotions and come to peace with the self- sabotaging beliefs I was holding close to my heart.

For the past twenty years, I have had the joy and pleasure of giving guidance, love, and support to women. If I help them, they too can be strong, fit, and healthy. They can be free from the emotional chains that keep them inside the walls of limiting beliefs, food addictions, gaining weight, and belly challenges.

I was compelled to use my knowledge to help others. But still, I had to stop and ask myself, "Why are you teaching this, Tina?" My belief system made me acknowledge that I was going through this for a good reason. **My sister's suffering, and my mess, was about to become my message…**

As a crusader for healthy, permanent weight loss, I just can't stand by any longer and watch another **charlatan promote another fad diet.** These diets are full of disease-causing chemicals that ruin people's metabolism and their lives. They teach things that just don't work. My mission is to save every woman that I can, and show them how to lose weight and keep it off forever without fad diets and gimmicks!

But before we move on, let's address an elephant in the room.

You may be thinking that you've tried all the diet's out there and there are none that work. That's the answer… I do not teach or coach a FAD diet. Instead, I teach a natural way to lose weight by **eating real yummy food without starving yourself**.

I do this by helping you understand why you are eating unhealthy things. The object is not to educate you on every aspect of the ever-changing landscape of diet and weight loss… Just your little piece of it!

Most importantly, When I work with you, we address the **emotional issues** behind the reasons you gained weight in the first place. Using techniques that work, I've been teaching people for many years how to release themselves from the bondage of their emotions; these emotions that keep them trapped and overeating.

Emotions and stress eating are at the core of destructive yo-yo dieting. **As published by the Harvard Medical School in July 2018, they showed how obesity was associated with emotional eating and stress, and that the way to reverse it is through meditation, exercise, and social support which are all part of this program.**

When you join forces with me, it will be the last weight loss program you will ever have to be in. I hold your hand throughout and show you the way. I believe in you and I know you CAN do this and get *Finally Thin Forever.*

Let me tell you another story…

When I was in my thirties, I worked for a chiropractor and she taught nutrition to her patients. I stayed late for each and every workshop, soaking up every bit of information that I could. She always spoke of going on a detox where you simply don't eat for three days and drink this crazy apple cider vinegar drink and cayenne pepper. Who does that and survives?

It took me three years before I would even think of doing a detox and now I teach my clients the easy way to detox their bodies with real whole foods, not by starving themselves.

Fast forward from this experience, I realized that I had some serious emotional issues and I was using food to stuff them down and keep them hidden, even from myself. I was afraid of having hunger pangs, and not having food nearby. This, I believe, came from being anorexic as a child as well as my experience in a subway station. Let me explain...

One day, at the end of summer, I was in France. I was coming home after guiding bike trips throughout the country. I was in the subway early in the morning and found myself dragging my heavy bag full of gifts to take home to my family. It was heavy, I hadn't eaten breakfast, and I walked for what seemed like miles. Occasionally, folks came by, felt sorry for me, and helped me drag my bag through the long hallways and up or down steps of the subway.

Finally, I arrived at the subway car... exhausted and drenched in sweat. Before I knew it, I was blacking out. Yup, that's right. I passed out in the subway station all by myself. I came around within a few seconds. I was completely flushed and a bit scared. I ate a banana I had with me, and felt better.

What did I learn? That I had low blood sugar (hypoglycemia) from not eating breakfast and from eating a carb-loaded dinner the night before. At the time, I was also a very heavy carb eating vegetarian. I simply didn't know better. I also learned that being hypoglycemic was not a death sentence and can easily be reversed.

Throughout my life, I've had a morphed vision of my body. I always thought that I was fat and typically wore clothes that were too big for me. Mind you, in my twenties, I only weighed 120 pounds at 5'4." But, I was never satisfied. I realize now that I was hiding. If I had to put my finger on what I was hiding from, I couldn't tell you specifically. But, I can guess that I was hiding from sexual attention from guys. I found the attention uncomfortable and even writing about it now is not easy.

I was always exercising excessively or dieting to get rid of the weight and then hiding it with clothes. I know that it sounds incredibly silly, but that was how my brain was wired. I now know there is a term for this, and it is called, "Body Dysmorphia".

Over the past ten years, I have been practicing modalities to help overcome emotional eating, which I teach to my clients. The most powerful modality is called the peace process. Using this process, you can go from having a super-strong feeling on anything, such as cupcakes or pizza. It might even be a current negative event. We move to a mindset where we are neutral about it. Sometimes it occurs within minutes, and sometimes it takes a few sessions. Think of Layers, it's all about peeling off the layers. I found out that I have the ability to hold space for my clients... to allow them to heal themselves from traumatic events without even having to think about those events.

In December of 2019, I became certified as a peace process practitioner and also earned the distinction of mastery in instant miracles. Yes, I'm certified and know that I don't heal people, they heal themselves, I simply hold the space for them.

I can now say that I no longer have a morphed vision of my body. I fully and completely accept my body for the gift that it is. Yes, even every fat cell (that mostly accumulates in my inner thighs and my boobs)! I love those especially because they are what makes up the most special and beautiful person in my life...me!

Yes, I eat healthy meals. I cheat every once in a while (especially ice cream when we go to the beach). I exercise to have fun not because I have to. I have surrendered to being 53 and going through perimenopause with wonky periods, hot flashes in the middle of the night, heavy bleeding out of nowhere... all of it! I absolutely love my body and love who I have become in my life. My work is one of passion and love for all women who are on the same journey as me and want support to live healthy, vibrant, and free for the rest of their lives.

You too can heal from the past and love your body. Yes, every inch of it!

So much love to you and humongous hugs (I love hugs).

Tina "I Love you, I Believe In You" McDermott

If you are ready to take your life to a new level and want to learn the secrets to weight loss, download my free EBOOK: The Joyful Gut Reboot. www.tinamcdermott.com/JG

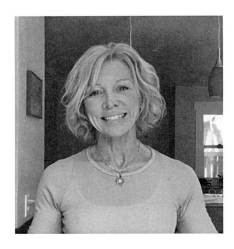

Catherine Ebeling

Enthralled with an insatiable zest for life, Catherine is the personifi-cation of what it means to turn misfortune into fortune. At the age of 50, Cat struggled through menopause while suffering a devastating financial loss and the breakup of her 20 year marriage. She decided to turn her life around by also walking away from an unfulfilling job and embark on the career of her dreams. Knowing that diseases start with bad eating habits, Cat became a student of nutrition. Earning her Bachelor's degree and Masters of Science in Nursing-Public Health, Cat wrote her first book, "The Fat Burning Kitchen" which instantly became a best-seller. She has subsequently written "The Top 101 Foods That Fight Aging", "The Diabetes Fix", and "Healthy Foods Made Easy".

She believes that enjoying life to the fullest means adopting a consistent healthy lifestyle that includes a healthy diet, regular exercise, a great social network and a positive mindset. It's NEVER too late to start anew. Menopause can be a journey of self-discovery, self-love and amazing experiences. Cat practices what she preaches and for her, life is just beginning.

NATURAL SOLUTIONS TO BALANCE HORMONES AND EASE MENOPAUSE SYMPTOMS

By Catherine Ebeling

IT WAS A BEAUTIFUL, hot, sunny summer day in 2007. I turned my brand new SUV into our private drive marked by stone lions guarding the entrance. I drove up to my gorgeous, custom-built home sitting on a wooded hillside with amazing views. I hit the garage door opener and pulled inside the three-car garage. I was alone, having dropped my three kids off at their friends' house for a while. I closed the garage door, got out of the car, and collapsed on the steps in the garage, sobbing so hard I couldn't stop. My world was totally falling to pieces and I didn't know what to do.

Our finances were a mess, and we were sinking deeper into debt while my husband's real estate venture crashed and burned. My marriage was falling apart—harsh words, negativity and anger filled the air. I hated my job as a hospital nurse, but now did not seem like the time to make career changes. I felt like I had fallen into a black hole and could not climb out, no matter how hard I tried. Oh, and I was going through menopause too, as I soon found out.

I dreaded every night, knowing it would be long hours in the dark–tossing and turning. Anxiety attacks filled my days, along with mood swings, depression, tears, forgetfulness, loss of energy, horrible PMS and unpredictable periods. One month my periods were barely there, and then two weeks later, I'd have such a heavy flow, I couldn't leave the house.

I prayed for answers. I found a job working at a physician's practice that specialized in wellness, anti-aging and, bioidentical hormone therapy. I enjoyed working in spite of still struggling through all the hormonal symptoms. The worst was not sleeping and the anxiety attacks. They would strike out of nowhere, even while driving.

One day, I was chatting with the doctors in my practice and mentioned how I just couldn't sleep. I had tried melatonin, magnesium and even a few prescription medications which had had terrible side effects. One of the doctors asked me how old I was. I told him, "Fifty". He said, "We should have your hormone levels checked, I bet you are going through menopause."

I was stunned. I had no idea. In the midst of the turmoil of my life, I never put two and two together to realize that many of my issues were hormone-related. I was actually starting to believe my soon-to-be-ex-husband's opinion that I was 'crazy'.

I got lab work done for estrogen, progesterone, testosterone, and FSH. My doctor took one look at my lab work and told me my hormones were basically at zero, except for FSH, indicating I was in the throes of menopause. He said, "It's no wonder you feel like you do." That comment was actually a relief—and validation.

Now I knew there was a path forward. I could actually begin climbing my way out of the black hole of my life. Perhaps I wasn't actually 'crazy' after all.

My doctor started me on some progesterone to help control some of the initial menopause symptoms I was experiencing. The progesterone was a blessed relief. I started sleeping well for the first time in months, and the anxiety just stopped. So did many of my other symptoms like the hot flashes and the mood swings. I felt calm and happy again. It was amazing. I began thinking I could move forward with my life and that positive changes may be in my future.

I spent a couple years working for the medical practice and learned quite a bit about hormone fluctuations, pre-menopause, peri-menopause and menopause. I counseled many patients and helped them ease their symptoms and get their lives back. I watched so many patients go from sullen and miserable, to upbeat and on top of the world. It was truly an eye-opening and rewarding experience.

Why Do Hormones Matter?

Proper hormonal balance can change your outlook, your health, and the entire trajectory of your life. Hormones most definitely have an effect on us—physically, mentally, and emotionally.

Hormones for women include more than the sex hormones of estrogen, progesterone and testosterone. Our bodies function optimally with a delicate balance of sex hormones, thyroid hormones, leptin, insulin, cortisol, growth hormone, serotonin, melatonin and more.

When any one hormone level goes up or down, it can wreak havoc on all the other hormones. So instead of a symphony of hormones working together, out of whack hormones can become just a cacophony of noise. And that's when we get all those hormonal symptoms.

Hormones can affect almost every function in our body. Hormones play a part in our hunger or satisfaction, how well we sleep, how we react to stress, how we respond to exercise, how we metabolize our food, our sex drive, our moods, our energy levels and how quickly we age. And, hormones have a lot to do with our feelings of self-confidence and overall wellbeing.

Signs that Your Hormones May be Out of Balance

- ► Weight gain—especially around the middle
- ► Low thyroid symptoms
- ► Mood changes and emotional lability
- ► Anxiety and depression
- ► Endometriosis
- ► PMS
- ► Breast tenderness
- ► Insomnia
- ► Irritability
- ► Loss of interest in sex
- ► Fatigue

► Hot flashes

► Hair loss or hair growth in unusual places

► Blood sugar instability

► Food cravings

► Lack of passion and drive

► Fluid retention

► Headaches/Migraines

How Estrogen Contributes to Heath Issues

Estrogen is the hormone that makes us 'female' and is responsible for our female characteristics such as breast development, menstrual periods, and the tendency to store fat around our hips. Estrogen surges at adolescence and begins its decline in our forties.

Estrogen comes in different forms—estradiol, estrone and estriol. Each of these have different roles in our bodies. Estrogen is produced by the ovaries pre-menopause, produced in large quantities by the placenta during pregnancy, and even after menopause we still produce small amounts of estrone in the adrenals and body fat. The more body fat a woman has, the more estrogen is produced.

Estrogen is responsible for causing weight gain, especially around the hips and breasts during pregnancy. It is estrogen's job to ensure that our bodies can support a pregnancy even through a famine. Estrogen also causes fluid retention and can be pro-cancerous.

What is Estrogen Dominance?

Estrogen dominance is a condition that occurs when our estrogen levels are too high in relation to progesterone. This can be characterized by symptoms such as breast tenderness or fibrocystic breasts, premenstrual syndrome, mood swings, decreased sex drive, uterine fibroids, and weight gain. Estrogen dominance also dramatically raises the risk of ovarian cancer and breast cancer. Estrogen dominance can also contribute to depression, headaches, infertility, insomnia, thyroid dysfunction and water retention. Estrogen dominance is present in the majority of women in their 40's and 50's.

What Causes Estrogen Dominance?

► Conventional hormone therapy with synthetic estrogen, or contraceptive pill

► Exposure to xenoestrogens (artificial estrogens in our environment)

► Weight gain

► Hysterectomy

► Declining progesterone levels (often begins after age of thirty-five)

► Peri-menopause

► Menopause

► Diet and inflammation

As we age, progesterone levels tend to drop fairly quickly after the age of 35 or so. By the time we reach menopause, our progesterone has hit rock bottom, while estrogen is still in a gradual decline. Due to diet and lifestyle factors, most women in American tend to have estrogen levels approximately twice as high as they naturally should be.

Many of the peri-menopause and menopause symptoms we attribute to lack of estrogen are actually from low levels of progesterone. Estrogen and progesterone need to exist in a particular ratio—generally 1:100 estrogen-progesterone.

In fact, at menopause, progesterone decreases to about $1/120^{th}$ of our premenstrual levels, while estrogen only decreases by about ½. While conventional thinking is that we have too little estrogen by the time we reach menopause, in fact, most women have *too much* estrogen in relationship to progesterone.

In less industrialized countries, women who eat a primitive diet consisting of large amounts of vegetables, whole grains and naturally raised protein have far lower levels of estrogen. Not surprisingly, women from these cultures do not report difficulties with menopause or peri-menopause.

Fiber in the diet also helps to clear the body of excess estrogen by carrying it out in bowel movements. Circulating estrogen is sent to the liver to be processed, and then sent to the large intestine to be eliminated. If there is not enough fiber in a woman's diet to carry out the estrogen, estrogen gets reabsorbed. So consequently, a diet high in fiber is helpful to balance out estrogen dominance.

What about Xenoestrogens?

Let's talk briefly about xenoestrogens. Xenoestrogens are artificial, chemically-produced estrogens. Xenoestrogens are far more potent and dangerous to our health than natural estrogens. Xenoestrogens compete at the same receptor sites in our bodies as our natural hormones and can easily cause estrogen dominance. In fact, xenoestrogens are powerful enough to affect even men. Ever seen a man with 'man boobs'? This is the effect of xenoestrogens. Xenoestrogens can dramatically increase cancer risk (for men or women) as well as estrogen dominance.

Where do xenoestrogens come from? Unfortunately, they are all around us. Xenoestrogens are in pesticides, herbicides, our food supply, birth control, car and truck exhaust, nail polish, cosmetics, toiletries, shampoos, dry cleaning chemicals, and nearly all plastics. However, you can minimize the effects of xenoestrogens by being aware of them and making changes in lifestyle, diet and personal care products.

What About Progesterone?

Progesterone is what we call a 'master hormone'. It is essential as a building block for our other hormones. Even men require small amounts of progesterone as a precursor to testosterone. Progesterone is made by our ovaries. Progesterone for women serves as a balancing hormone to estrogen and offsets the risks of too much estrogen.

When progesterone levels plummet in a woman's forties, supplemental progesterone can actually help to reduce many of the symptoms of estrogen dominance. But that's not all, progesterone can have far-reaching benefits for the whole body. Other benefits of progesterone include:

- ▶ Reduces painful ovarian cysts
- ▶ Prevents uterine cancer, breast cancer
- ▶ Lessen the chances of ovarian cysts
- ▶ Prevent or mitigate PMS, especially during perimenopause
- ▶ Stimulates bone formation
- ▶ Helps prevent autoimmune disease
- ▶ Improves estrogen receptor sensitivity
- ▶ Prevents arterial plaque and prevents heart disease and strokes
- ▶ Lessens fibrocystic breast issues
- ▶ Aids the body in metabolizing fat
- ▶ Gets rid of excess stored fluids
- ▶ Increases GABA in brain and drastically reduces anxiety
- ▶ Antidepressant
- ▶ Facilitates deeper, more restful sleep
- ▶ Helps balance and normalize thyroid function
- ▶ Normalizes and balances blood sugar
- ▶ Protects against blood clots
- ▶ Helps with weight loss
- ▶ Restores cells' oxygen supply
- ▶ Protects the brain from injury after strokes or traumatic brain injuries
- ▶ Important for repair of nerves, especially the myelin sheath (MS)

Is it any wonder we have noticeable symptoms when progesterone drops?

The Dance of Hormones

Our bodies also create other hormones including:

- ▶ DHEA-made by the adrenal glands, and a precursor to testosterone, estrogen and some progesterone. DHEA peaks at age 25 then declines. We need it to help fight aging.

- ▶ Testosterone-made by the ovaries and adrenal glands. Helps burn fat, build muscle, create stronger bones and adds to motivation, energy and a sense of wellbeing

- ▶ Cortisol-Made by the adrenals and also from progesterone. Helps us manage stress, maintains blood sugar, and metabolize nutrients. Too much cortisol (usually from stress) can cause weight gain, sleeplessness, other health problems. A progesterone imbalance causes problems with cortisol. Low cortisol also equals poor thyroid function.

Chronic stress can affect many bodily systems and can wreak havoc on hormone balance. Chronic stress can make you feel exhausted and 'out of gas'. Stress can affect insulin, progesterone, estrogen, testosterone, thyroid, melatonin and cortisol levels. Nothing in the body works as it should with high levels of stress.

Estrogen, Progesterone and Thyroid Hormones

The thyroid hormone regulates metabolism. A low thyroid or hypothyroid can cause you to gain weight, have low energy, hair and nails grow slowly, intolerance to cold, and low immune function. A hyperthyroid causes high metabolism, weight loss, hair loss, sleeplessness, and anxiety.

Women with estrogen dominance and low progesterone often have symptoms of low thyroid—even if thyroid lab work shows up normal. Other issues that interfere with thyroid function include high cortisol levels and gluten intolerance.

Thyroid hormones include T3 and T4. T3 is the active form of thyroid hormone in the body. If your body is not efficient at converting T4 into T3 you can have low thyroid, but it may not even show up on a standard thyroid test. Many physicians never check this part of thyroid function, but it is essential. If the thyroid is not functioning optimally, cortisol, estrogen and progesterone may be low as well.

Inflammation and Hormones

Many people have chronic inflammation due to poor diet, too much sugar, food sensitivities, toxins in the environment, high stress, and lack of sleep. Chronic inflammation can show up in many different forms including: Belly fat, chronic pain, accelerated aging, food allergies, blood sugar problems, autoimmunity, IBS and other inflammatory bowel diseases, cardiovascular disease, cancer, skin problems and hormone imbalances—especially thyroid hormones, estrogen and progesterone.

Inflammation levels can be tested by looking at C-Reactive protein (CRP), blood sugar levels (HbA1c), erythrocyte sedimentation rate (ESR), and plasma viscosity (PV).

However, our hormones are at their highest levels in the mid-twenties and as they decrease, inflammation levels also tend to rise. Hormone treatment in the proper balance can reduce inflammation.

How Do We Lower Inflammation?

These steps can help lower inflammation:

1. First eliminate inflammatory foods along with strategic detoxes that clear excess hormone levels from the body, stop food sensitivities, and clear hormone receptors.

2. Avoid dangerous hormone-disrupting artificial estrogens in the environment by avoiding particular home cleaning supplies, laundry soaps, dry cleaning, toiletries, makeup, shampoos, pesticides and other chemical-based products.

3. Practice good self-care to lower stress such as meditation, good sleep and exercise.

Fixing Estrogen Dominance and Balancing Hormones

There is an easy system to rebalance your hormones and get your estrogen and progesterone back into balance. In the process, you will lose weight, sleep better, feel better, eliminate anxiety, and also get rid of many of those unpleasant menopause or peri-menopause symptoms. Making changes in diet, weight loss, removal of xenoestrogens and lowering inflammation will help you regain hormone balance— perhaps even better than ever!

I offer a 90 Day Health & Hormone Fix to help you balance your hormones and feel younger, stronger and sexier. This is a full recipe to help you:

- ► Lose weight/reset your body composition
- ► Rebalance your hormones
- ► Detox your system and reduce inflammation
- ► Stop or slow down chronic disease
- ► Regain your energy, vitality, and passion for living and loving
- ► Gain a mindset of empowerment and self-confidence
- ► Turn back the clock to look and feel younger

This wholistic, proven approach is based on groundbreaking, proven medical research from well-known doctors including Christine Northrup MD, Sara Gottfried MD, John Lee MD, Neal Barnard MD, Christine Robins, MD, and Stephanie Faubion MD–as well as my own 30+ years studying diet and health.

The 90-Day Health & Hormone Fix is Founded on 3 Pillars

- ► **Reset**

    Through a supervised detox and reset diet, we determine which foods are causing inflammation, food sensitivities, gut dysbiosis, weight gain, and hormone imbalances.

► **Rebuild**

By analyzing your diet, looking at lab work, and gathering extensive health history, we develop a customized plan that works specifically for you–with proven diet, exercise, mindset, supplements, and lifestyle changes.

► **Rebalance**

By nourishing your body, mind and spirit with the foods it needs, we bring back into balance estrogen, progesterone, thyroid, insulin, cortisol, and testosterone, to bring back optimal health, optimal weight and optimal energy—along with new habits and knowledge to keep this balance for a lifetime.

Are you ready for lasting change?

► 90 days individualized health coaching by an RN/MSN who specializes in diet, health and hormone issues.

► Easy-to-use diet/food tracking app to track your intake, see your macros, balance your diet.

► 12 weeks of multiple online educational modules consisting of videos, workouts, mindset work, recipes, meal plans and more.

The Rest of My Story

I literally walked out of an awful job one day—not knowing what the next day would bring. I got divorced and found MYSELF again. I actually sailed through menopause smoothly and with ease, once I knew what to do.

I got in better shape, found a new group of positive, upbeat friends, ended up in the dream career I always wanted, and moved to a town where I'd always wanted to live. And I found the love of my life!

The transition through menopause can actually become a catalyst for much upheaval in one's life. Suddenly things that you were content with no longer work for you. You start thinking of yourself and putting yourself first. Stopping the distraction of unpleasant hormonal symptoms, getting your health on track, and stepping into a positive, 'can-do' mindset can help you create the life of your dreams.

I never regret the decisions I have made or the path I took, and I am forever grateful for the changes that menopause brought about. Was it Worth it? YES!!

My name is Catherine Ebeling. I am an RN with a Masters of Science in Nursing and Public Health and I am here to help you through this.

I have been studying diet, fitness and health for the past 30+ years–in addition to my clinical nursing experience, which includes anti-aging, preventative and regenerative medicine and bioidentical hormone therapy. I have had a life-long fascination with diet, fitness and nutrition that actually started while I was still in high school, when I started reading books by the world-famous nutritionist, Adele Davis.

I realized that we, as humans, have the ultimate power over our bodies and our health by what we put into them. Wanting to learn even more about human biology, nutrition, health and disease, I went back to school to study for a BSN in nursing. I just recently completed my Masters of Science in Nursing (at age 60). I've written six books on diet and health that have sold hundreds of thousands of copies all over the world. I am an expert on diet and health and want to share that knowledge with you.

You can do anything–at ANY age! It's never too late to start! Don't be ashamed to be a late bloomer! You can blossom when everyone else is wilting! Here are a few other things I've done since the age of 50…

- ► Winning a regional bike race against 50 of the top women's racers in the country
- ► Exciting Class 5 white water rafting in Peru, Costa Rica, Nepal, Ecuador, New Zealand, Scotland, Zambia, Utah and Colorado.
- ► Exploring the jungles of Costa Rica, Nicaragua and Columbia.
- ► Landing at the world's most dangerous airport Lukla, Nepal to hike the Himalayas.

- ► Wild animal safaris in Botswana and Zimbabwe.
- ► SCUBA diving in the Mediterranean, Thailand, Costa Rica and Belize.
- ► Exploring the unspoiled beauty and wild animals of Galapagos
- ► Being guests of a tribe of indigenous locals in highlands of Peru
- ► Walking the Great Wall of China
- ► Hiking the Grand Canyon rim to rim

When I am not traveling, I live in Boulder, Colorado at the base of the beautiful Rocky Mountains where I ride my bike or run up into the mountains every day that I can.

This should be the BEST chapter of your life and I want to help you to live your best life ever!

Let's discuss ways that we can get you on the path to all the best things in your life: health, happiness, fulfillment and love. I am here to give you the tools, the support and the roadmap you need.

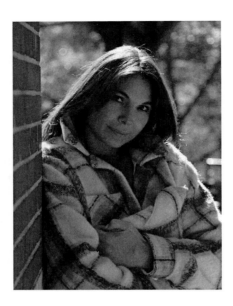

Nadiya Williams

Nadiya is the epitome of "a quiet strength." She is an intimate fitness instructor and reiki healer from the Ukraine. A breast cancer survivor that left her struggling with self doubt and lack of self-confidence, she felt her femininity slipping away. She needed a way to believe in herself again, to reawaken her sensuality and to recover the many pleasures of being a woman. Thus the birth of Feminine Revival.

Feminine Revival brings a new and renewed level of fulfillment to women, helping them to reconnect with their essential femininity. This is now Nadiya's life's work and she feels honored to share something powerful and life enhancing to women.

Nadiya is an expert in IMbuilding. This is not just a technique for training women's most intimate muscles, but her whole body. With daily practice, the body responds to IMbuliding very quickly awakening the desires for sensuality, sex and love.

Knowing Nadiya is knowing true femininity. With class and finesse, she lovingly leads women from feeling useless to a place of empowerment. She is the manifestation of what she teaches.

SECRETS ABOUT FEMALE SEXUALITY

By Nadiya Williams

I AM BROKEN. I FEEL NOTHING down there. I no longer get aroused. I don't like my body and I am uncomfortable undressing in front of my partner. My femininity has disappeared. My inner woman is dead. I can come up with 100 reasons not to make love with my husband. Where has my sexuality gone? What is it? Do any of these phrases resonate with you?

Some years ago, I was afraid to even ask myself these questions. Why? I was afraid that I didn't have the answers. I can blame everything and everyone for my breast cancer, unsuccessful fertility treatments, painful divorce, and beginning stages of menopause. There were several treatments, and I didn't have the power to handle all of the obstacles thrown my way. I had so many feelings, but none about femininity or sexuality. I think I buried them, until I was prescribed antidepressant pills.

And here, the story begins.

I thought about other solutions. How can I heal my soul, my body, and get back to the woman I knew before and return even better?

I decided not to take the antidepressant pills. Instead I began my daily rediscovery of everyday little pleasures. I decided to study female sexuality, talking to women and men to try and understand how they feel about their sexuality. I became an intimate pelvic muscle instructor simply because pills could not fix me.

Now, I love my work. I love helping women feel happier, healthier, sexier, confident and pleasurable.

My name is Nadiya Williams, and I am the founder of Feminine Revival, a place for women's rediscovery of the sensual self. Feminine Revival didn't just appear, it was the revival of my femininity... a reawakening of sexual energy that I'd lost a long time ago. It was my holistic approach to heal my body and my soul.

I was born and raised in the Ukraine during a Sovietunien regime. In 1991 I left the Ukraine for Paris, where I was a fashion model for 20 years. In 2009 I met my ex husband, fell in love like a teenage girl, and moved to New York City. I have no regrets as I look back on those years and my decision to leave everything behind. Even after going through my divorce later on, I am still grateful for all the experiences and new opportunities. But, I will be honest with all of the women reading this book. If my ex husband hadn't kicked me out of our bedroom I would not be here today.

I think being sexually refused by someone you love unconditionally is one of the worst feelings a woman or man can experience. You feel like the most lonely and invaluable person in the world.

Sex itself is very mechanical, and if your genitals are not working, it will not and cannot happen. However, this is okay because it's fixable. Yet, without touching, communication, and quality time you're left feeling unworthy, and this can bring you to a mentally unhealthy place. For me, this was a wake up call, and while taking a pill might have been an easier solution, I didn't.

Now I want to tell you all about the IMbuilding (intimate muscle building) program. The program helped me overcome all of my obstacles, and become even better in every way. Of course my painful separation impacted my confidence, but going through breast cancer and menopause at the same time also affected my health. My female parts became a little bit numb. I lost sensitivity, experienced hot flashes, stressed incontinence, a disturbing burning in the morning down there, and UTIs that drove me crazy. I felt like my entire body was falling apart.

Nevertheless, to enhance my pelvic floor I began Kegel exercises. Unfortunately these didn't help me too much because I was performing them incorrectly. In my search for alternate solutions on how to improve my intimate health, I came across the School of IMbuilding (intimate muscle building), and that was it.

I had nothing to lose so I signed up and dove right into the world of IMbuilding. It was eye-opening, enlightening and disarming all at the same time. Tears of accepting my body and understanding that at 47 years old, my mind and body were not living in harmony. I was sitting at the corner of the studio, watching other women do their exercises. Some of them brought their small children and others came with friends. I remember looking at their expressions, their smiles, and their body movements. The room was infused with warm feminine energy. This is something you can't touch, yet it engulfs and nourishes you. This energy permeates you from within and then radiates outward. The women were so open about their experiences, exchanging discoveries about their intimate health, and their body's new sensations. What a joy I had, I felt like I had returned to my homeland. I felt myself reconnecting with the world, to myself, to other people, and after just a week of taking classes, the world started feeling me too. That was it, the decision was made. I submitted documents to the original source of the International Federation School of IMbuilding. I studied, was assessed, and then I received my certificate.

My goal is to help women the same way I helped myself. I want to share this amazing knowledge with all women, and tell them that our pelvic floor is not just a part of our body. It's the source of a woman's power! Do you know where this is? It's in our second chakra. A sacred place where we create new life and plant the seeds of our child.

This power is so powerful, so fearless, and so magical. Unfortunately a lot of women don't understand this or were never taught about this source of power. Women have a storage where they collect layers after layers of trauma, pain, negative emotions, and sadness. We need to erase the trauma and negative emotions, and work on our inner woman. In my practice I see women transform everyday. When women are awakening their sexual energy they become more confident, happier, healthier, and sexier. And no one will disagree with the fact that women with these qualities are powerful in astonishing ways. She is more pleasant to be around and her source of power has no limits because she doesn't need to draw this energy from anyone. She needs no one to fulfill her needs because she has her feminine sexuality and her own well being. She radiates this to the world, her love, her motherhood, and her happiness.

The Eros energy is the source of the Magic's power.

Everyone has it! Men and Women have been given this beautiful gift by nature. It is in us, but because of different circumstances present in our everyday lives, such as religion, culture, and our family's approach to sex, a lot of us struggle with discovering our sexuality. However, the secret is simple: we need to awaken this life force energy, by connecting our mind and body. We must let ourselves enjoy simple daily pleasures by being attentive to our bodies. This means relishing in the flavors of delicious foods, feeling the sensations of soft sweaters on our skin, and having conversations about what we like, and what we don't like. Yes, sometimes to reach the point of ultimate pleasure we need to experience painful emotions. Talking to other women and asking them questions about sexuality definitely helps, but we must discover what we need for ourselves. I always ask my students why they're in my class. It's important to understand what you need to rediscover in yourself. For me, it is easier to approach my clients knowing that I can help them gain the results they desire.

I always begin my program by explaining a woman's pelvic anatomy. Having knowledge on how your body functions is key to controlling certain parts of it. Some parts of women's pelvic intimate muscles can be controlled voluntarily. I am always surprised by the fact that 70% of women know nothing about their genitals or how they function. How can we achieve pleasure if we don't know anything about our precious parts? Don't get me wrong, there are numerous different ways to feel pleasure in the world, because enjoying ice cream can be considered a pleasure too. However, I am talking about your feminine, intimate pleasure. The feeling of being sexually desirable and sexually satisfied. I believe sexual energy is connected to a woman's pelvic area. Hundreds of years ago, women who were deemed too sexual were burned at the stake. They were considered witches because they had too much power. Not much has changed since those days. We still have our power and we will always have it. So, let's use it to benefit our health and pleasure. As I said already, knowledge of our body is the first step. Liking yourself and accepting the way you are is key. In my classes I first use breathing exercises to relax the body and pelvis. Then I explain to women how to work on their intimate parts.

I am helping women explore and develop their feminine sexuality, and enjoy intimacy in entirely new ways using the IMbuilding program through Feminine Revival. This program helps thousands of women awaken their sexuality naturally. I am teaching women about their body, and helping them train their intimate pelvic muscles. I believe this is the key to sexual satisfaction for them and their partner. This program is enhancing their overall health and sense of well being.

IMbuilding (intimate muscles building), is a personal fitness program developed for our pelvic floor and vaginal muscles. It allows every woman, regardless of age, to develop, strengthen, restore, and learn how to voluntarily control her most intimate muscles!

No one will argue with me, if I say that we need to use and train all the muscles in our body, because muscles feel best when they are at work. The muscles we don't use will atrophy sooner or later. In order to build muscles, we need to give them resistance! We do this in our program with the help of a patented, personal vaginal training device made from medical grade materials. We build muscles to support pelvic organs, and prevent prolapse and incontinence. We develop elasticity of our muscles to assist in many different functions, such as birth, urination, and sexual function. Lastly, we increase sensitivity of our nerve endings to enhance sexual pleasure.

By contracting and strengthening your intimate muscles you increase blood flow and lymphatic circulation to your whole pelvic floor area, as well as the supply of oxygen to your vaginal tissue. As you do exercises over time your strength will grow, the muscles of your pelvic floor will become broader and thicker, and you'll gain increased muscle tone. Your mucus membrane becomes more stretchy, releasing a lot of secretion.

Intimate fitness is not just Kegel exercises, it's personal training for your pelvic muscles, for ultimate pleasure and control. Our program has no limitations and is suitable for every woman. We can help young women develop self-confidence, awaken their sensitivity, decrease period pain, and gain sexual knowledge. We help prenatal and postpartum women facilitate childbirth and with post birth recovery of the pelvic floor. Lastly, we are here to help pre and post menopausal women rejuvenate post menopausal vaginal tissue.

The program also has several health and pleasure benefits. I always like to say "If you want to give pleasure, you must know pleasure!"

The pleasure benefits of IMbuilding include:

► Increased libido and sexual desire

► Increased feminine self-confidence

► Better and easier orgasms

► Lubrication and arousal during sex

► Stronger vaginal muscles for more powerful orgasms

► Development of erogenous zones

► Stronger bond with your partner

I also tell my students that "A healthy pelvic floor contributes to healthy sex, and healthy sex leads to a healthy life."

The health benefits of IMbulding include:

► Enhanced vaginal control

► Less painful periods

► Tightening and toning of vaginal canal

► Prevention of prolapse

► Improved bladder control, reduced involuntary urination

► Easier childbirth and postpartum recovery of vaginal tone

► Post-menopausal rejuvenation of vaginal tissue

Everything I am teaching I underwent myself, and learned from my student's feedback. Each of my students who completed the program became like sisters because female energy is such a powerful source of women friendship and empowerment. Here are a few testimonials from women who went through the program.

"I had a hard time connecting with my body. I felt disconnected and this is because when I was younger I experienced a sexually traumatic event. I didn't feel like my body belonged to me anymore.

When I first started taking the classes I didn't know if they'd work because I thought I was broken. I decided to give it a chance because I had heard so many great reviews from other women. I met Nadiya and she was so sweet. She showed me the anatomy of the pelvic floor and this was something that I had never learned before. In my culture, discussing this is a taboo.

After the first class I already felt this confidence and this energy. I felt so amazing after this first class that I decided I wanted to put in the work, because you have to put in work to see results. I have a three year old daughter so I'd find myself making time to practice in the shower and at work. Each class I learned new things and the breathing exercises really helped.

Through this program I learned how to use my body in a whole new way that I never knew before. By the final class I didn't feel broken anymore. I felt reconnected with my body, and this person that forced themselves on me all those years ago no longer has this power over me. It's my body now, this is me."

-Shanelle age 28

"Feminine revival has helped me discover and align my feminine energy. Before, my sexuality was scattered- I knew it was there but I never had a grasp on how to control and, especially, appreciate it.

Once I started with Nadiya, I felt results instantly. I took the class with my best friend and when we left, we both felt different, but in the best way possible. We felt our sacral chakra awaken.

Since then, I've kept practicing and have benefited immensely. Masturbation has become a beautiful ritual, not something I was embarrassed about. The strength of my orgasm makes me feel so amazing. My imagination has no limits and I have never felt so free in my own skin.

Unlocking my sacral chakra has made me see myself in a new light. These classes gave me the feminine strength I needed to get off all of my pills (antidepressants and birth control) and live a beautiful and grateful life.

Forever grateful for Nadiya and her practice."

-Sofia age 22

"When I first started taking classes with Nadiya I wasn't sure what to expect. I didn't necessarily have anything that I wanted to work on or fix, but after our first session I felt different. I felt energized and I felt a kind of sexual energy that I have never felt before.

After our second session and a few hours of practicing on my own (yes you have to do the homework to see results) my partner even noticed a difference. He saw my confidence grow and this came from my ability to control my intimate muscles. I was able to control the pace of sex and this was something I had never done before. However, it helped us reach another level of intimacy that we hadn't experienced with each other. This definitely improved our sex life!!

But, I will have to say that I saw my biggest result after just 3 months of training. I was always someone who had extremely painful period cramps and a heavy cycle. I started taking birth control because of this, and while the medication helped with my heavy flow, it didn't do much for my cramps. After completing Feminine Revival's program and training consistently a few times a week, my cramps have almost completely disappeared. My period used to last a solid 5 to 7 days, and now it only lasts 3 days!

This has been huge for me and I think the beauty of Feminine Revival is that it can help women in so many different ways. The program helped me with my cramps and gain confidence with my partner, and on the flip side it helped one of my best friends awaken her sexuality and see herself in a new light. I believe Feminine Revival can help all women discover and reconnect with themselves in a way that they haven't before. I'm forever grateful to Nadiya for helping me and all the amazing work that she is doing for women."

-Izabela age 21

"My confidence in myself and in the bedroom is through the roof. In addition to now having painless periods, I also feel more energized, less stressed, more motivated and so much sexier. Feminine Revival has been a total revelation."

-Camilla age 27

"As one of the first participants of Feminine Revival in NYC, I'm happy and proud of my achievement working with Nadiya who is the most dedicated and passionate instructor you'll ever want to meet. My goal was getting back the sexuality and desire I had before my 3 kids. Already, after the second class, I began to feel the desire that I was missing... and from that day I didn't stop. I'm feeling happier inside and out! Thank you Nadiya!"

-Svetlana age 45

"I started IMbuilding training with Nadiya and literally after three classes I felt my libido start to wake up. I have more energy and during my periods, the cramps, which used to be terrible, have disappeared. I am confident and healthier than ever."

- Olga age 31

These are just a few of the beautiful testimonies from my Students. Unfortunately due to the current state of the world I haven't been able to train as many women in person. However, this period of self isolation inspired me to create an online course program for Feminine revival. Initially I tried guiding a few international groups of women via zoom, and their results were amazing. Eventually several women from other states began asking if I could do something online so they can exercise from the privacy of their home. This online program includes everything I teach my students in person, and more! I think it's important that all women all over the world have the opportunity to improve their intimate health. You should also have the option to train where you're most comfortable, because if you're comfortable you'll have better results, and my goal is to leave you feeling happier, healthier, sexier, and confident.

I worked on this program with my gynecologist, Dr. Lana Selitsky. She also took my classes and saw amazing results, improving both her health and intimate life. Nonetheless the online program truly has no limitations, and any woman can use this course to discover or rediscover some part of herself.

In this program women will learn how to do self exams. This is an amazing practice that helps women really understand how to control their pelvic floor muscles. The best thing a woman can do for herself is to take the time to learn about her female anatomy. This is why both the self exam video and the intimate massage video are crucial for our online course. The intimate massage is the key to awakening dormant and undeveloped nerve endings in our genitals and vagina. This is great for the pre and post menopause stage because the massage helps bring more blood flow and prevent atrophy of the vaginal mucous membranes. The program also includes several classes with exercises for relaxation and strengthening the pelvic floor. The exercises are perfect because women can perform them in their everyday activities. Every woman who completes the program will see a dramatic change in her health and her intimate life. The only condition is that you must practice to see results!

As I stated earlier, IMbuilding (intimate muscles building) helped me overcome many unpleasant symptoms produced by menopause and my breast cancer treatments. Although I've already mentioned this, I will repeat myself again and say that Menopause is not a problem. It's just a new stage of our lives and we simply have to learn how to dance with it. Of course the hormone levels and our bodies are both changing, but what I noticed with myself is that we are still the same women. It's our responsibility to take care of our bodies, our minds and to do what we can to keep the crazy hormones in harmony.

Breast cancer has enabled me from taking any hormone replace-ments, so I've learned how to deal with all my symptoms naturally. I found that yoga, particularly pranayama breathing helped me enor-mously with my hot flashes. My stress incontinence disappeared in 3 weeks after I did this program. The breath work combined with all of the squeezing and lifting of my pelvic floor muscles was extremely beneficial for me. All of this exercise brought a lot of blood flow to my pelvic area. This has helped me with my vaginal dryness, as well as using some creams made from natural ingredients. The numb-ness I felt disappeared, and my sensitivity increased and even became better than before.

As I mentioned earlier, when we empty the negativity, sadness, and unspoken conversations from our storage, we make room for the Eros energy, letting it flow throughout our body. When we establish a mind and body connection, changes happen and everyone experiences these differently. Since I dove into this powerful Eros energy, I discovered parts of myself that I never knew existed. I became a reiki healer, I learned Qigong (an ancient energy practice), and I started writing poetry.

To all of the beautiful women reading this, I want to tell you to love yourself and evaluate yourself. Even if you are in a great state and place in your life, know that there's always room for evaluating. One last thing, intimate fitness is not just about your muscles, it's all about you and accepting yourself. Remember how strong and beautiful you are, and know that the power you hold comes from within.

With all my love,
Nadiya Williams
www.femininerevival.com
Email: info@femininerevival.com
Instagram: @feminine_revival
Facebook: @feminine.revival

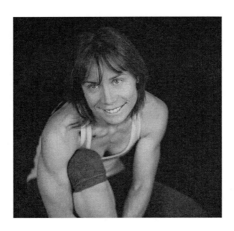

Jacqueline Martin

Jacqueline's beauty radiates from the inside out. Plagued by the former demons of body dysmorphia, Jacqueline chose to overcome this plight and thrive. Her early career launched as a professional triathlete in Canada. This morphed into her passion for pilates. Based in Poland, she developed her own signature pilates program that has been indoctrinated into "The Work' program originally developed by Joe Pilates. She is a frequent contributor and the developer of an exclusive lineage pilates training program at the Sense Studio in Warsaw. Her work has been featured in Vogue magazine.

Her most recent focus has been to develop a functional fitness program through the system of pilates to help women over forty. Jacqueline believes that bringing pilates to menopausal women benefits their overall health and enhances their physical and emotional wellbeing. As a 54 year old menopausal woman, she now enjoys optimal health. Her physical body emanates this transformation as well and she is vehement to share her discovery with women of the world.

HOW PILATES CHANGED MY LIFE?

By Jacqueline Martin

ONE MORNING IN 1952, way before I came into this world, my dad woke up and decided to buy a one-way ticket to Africa. He just followed his heart and never looked back. He settled in Abidjan (Ivory Coast), working as the top manager of Caterpillar Inc. Yet, his real passion was rescuing wild animals from poachers. His first rescue was an orphan leopard, which my father later named Bea. That extraordinary bond had lasted for five years before he released Bea in the wilderness, where she survived and started her own family. People used to call my father the animal whisperer, and very soon, many other wild cats found shelter on his farm. In 1956 he caught malaria and was taken to Montreal hospital where my mom was working as a nurse. He dated many ladies but still had his eyes on my mother. Unluckily, she would consistently refuse to go out with him.

After his release from the hospital, he stayed in Montreal for longer and rented an apartment. Only that way, he could still fight for my mother's attention. Six months later, they got married and flew back to Africa, where I came to the world in January of 1966. I was born a blue baby[1] after my mother had six miscarriages. The doctors told her that it was her last pregnancy. Yet, due to her profession, she truly believed in my survival. She ordered the doctors to have me in the incubator, where I thankfully started breathing. My first emotion

---

[1] A baby who is cyanotic (blue), usually due to a heart malformation that prevents the baby's blood from being fully oxygenated.

on this earth was fear, not love. I would rather be back in heaven than on this earth but my upbringing changed everything. Wild animals surrounded me at every turn. One of them was a chimpanzee that I named Catherine. I could not come near the wild cats, so she became my best friend. Like my dad and Bea, we created a unique bond between humans and animals.

My whole world was Catherine and the mixed school I went to as my parents did not believe in the racial divide. My dad took me to many dangerous places to show me villages ravaged by tribes. He was helping to rebuild it. He wanted to give them hope for a real education system and a promising career one day. I have seen places affected by terrible poverty where children have nothing but a deflated soccer ball and missing limbs. Yet, they are still playing and smiling for what they have now. I felt safe amongst this chaos of life and death. There was no ego and no judgment; people were full of unconditional love and acceptance for who they were.

After seven years spent together, it was time to release Catherine into the wilds. Letting her go was the hardest thing I ever had to face. Each year we would visit the place where we let her loose. To my surprise, she would come with her family and was not afraid of showing her babies to us. I will never forget these moments since they made me the person I am today.

When I turned fourteen, the Caterpillar company changed its policies to restrict the hiring of colored workers. My dad did not agree with those new rules, and one night, a phone call at 2 a.m. changed our lives as we had only twenty-four hours to leave. Luckily, one year earlier we had released all the wild animals. With just one suitcase, we walked out and went to the airport. I was wondering what happened as my parents did not explain anything to me. "The less you know, the better", they said.

We flew to the south of France, Toulon, and lived there for five years. Then my dad decided to move to Vancouver - he wanted me to have a better life and better opportunities. I graduated from Carson Graham Secondary School and became a sought out personal trainer - swim instructor and fitness guru.

I taught thirty classes a week plus swimming lessons and personal training. I always knew I would be in the fitness industry as I love helping people. Thanks to my passion, I met my future husband and we got married the following year. We moved to Nanaimo, a city on the east coast of Vancouver Island, where I decided to take nursing studies at Malaspina College. At the same time, I was maintaining my fitness life. I also bought a 30-acre farm.

Although having a career was my priority, I was still searching for who I am and what I want. After watching the movie *Terminator*, I fell in love with the biceps of Linda Hamilton. I joined a gym and nine months later, I entered my first middleweight British Columbia Championship competition and won my division.

Falling out of love with my husband, I found love in the gym, working out, and transforming my body. Besides the pleasure of training, I also liked the attention of Robin, one of the gym members.

After falling head over heels for him, I had an affair that lasted a few months until my husband finally found out. We divorced one year later. I will never forget the pain in his eyes. I hurt and crushed his heart, yet I carried on with a fifteen-year common-law relationship with Robin. During this period of my life, I discovered triathlons, and a few months later, I turned pro after advice from top coaches. I have always been a gifted athlete with a big heart, not afraid of training hard to do my best, and to win. Ironman Triathlon[2] became my thing - I spent thirty hours of training weekly, away from my relationship. Soon, I realized that Robin was more of a brother than a future husband. He started joining me and made his debut in Ironman as well.

I decided to put my nursing studies on hold and follow my heart into my athletic professional life. I hired Bev, who was the head coach of the Ladysmith Orcas Swim Club[3]. I wanted her to help

---

[2] One of a series of long-distance triathlon races, consisting of a 2.4-mile swim, a 112-mile bicycle ride and a marathon 26.22-mile run.

[3] A non-profit society that promotes youth health and fitness through swimming.

me swim faster. I knew that she would improve my training and get me to where I needed to be. She knew human bodies like no one else. She was coaching me physically, mentally, emotionally, and spiritually. Very soon, I became a part of the Ladysmith swim club community. Bev had incorporated Pilates into her training program with phenomenal results. She recommended I do more Pilates exercises to balance and strengthen my body. At her suggestion, I started the Kids of Steel[4] group triathlon training with Pilates and worked with pretty much the whole swim team. Not only were they great swimmers but also excellent triathletes. My trainer knew me thoroughly and she soon became my full-time coach. I was practicing thirty-five hours a week: Pilates, swimming, a bike and run training, transition workout, brick workout plus nutrition, rest and recovery with a full-time schedule, and a 10-year plan. As I became a top contender, I devoted myself entirely to the sport and left my relationship behind.

After a severe injury that left me out of competition for nine months, my coach Bev advised me to continue with Pilates. This encouragement not only saved me from surgery but brought me a full recovery from my injury. When I retired from pro levels, I became depressed. She recommended me to take my Pilates training certification - the rest is history. I opened my first studio in Ladysmith in 2004. It was located behind the beanery, a popular coffee place for locals and tourists. I started with four lessons a week and soon grew to twenty-four sessions with 8-10 people in one class. I realized I need a bigger space and I asked the universe for it. The next day, one of my clients proposed renting the upstairs of the building she recently bought. I took my first loan to renovate the place. During those few months of opening my new space, the waiting list was full. I also rented some space to a great physio and installed an Infrared sauna. Spinning classes and yoga were also in my schedule since I took my training for these. At that time, I was still teaching other fitness modules and Pilates.

---

[4] Free training program that helps motivate children and their families to exercise.

After a fifteen-year relationship, I left to be on my own for the first time in my life. I was not afraid of 'not making it'. I had my studio in a stunning apartment overlooking the ocean in Ladysmith. I was forty-two years old at that time. On July 1, 2007, through a triathlete friend of mine, I met Dean, and in 2008 I moved back to Vancouver to be with him. When we settled there, I started looking for a classical studio and I walked into Beyond Pilates Studio two blocks from where I was living and met Noam Gagnon. He was a graduate of Boulder Pilates Center, and eventually, I was ready to develop my teaching skills and started his teacher training program based on classical Romana Kryzanowska certification. I taught at his studio for two years and finally found my passion. I was still teaching spinning and yoga and took up boxing training with Sebastian at Contenders Boxing Studio in downtown Vancouver. I loved boxing as it brought me closer to Joseph Pilates and his method.

As I gained knowledge and understanding of the Pilates technique, also known as 'contrology'[5], I realized that Joe, himself, was a boxer and used to train fighters. With this method, you work on every single muscle and, if done correctly and consistently, it helps you get through punches and life difficulties with more ease. "A man is as old as his spine", explained Joe, and he put the accent on stretching, bending, tensing the body muscles, and flexing them without ropes, weights, punching bags, or props. There is no weight to lift. Have you ever seen an animal lifting weights for fun or exercise? His technique keeps the body focused on the powerhouse[6]. It helps to maintain balance and provides support for the spine. The Pilates method is a system of exercises that teaches alignment of the spine with the awareness of the breath and strengthens the torso. In three words: strength, stretch, and control of the mind. The best part of the training is that Pilates keeps you young and brings 'the zest of life' back.

---

[5] A complete coordination of body, mind, and spirit.
[6] The term created by Joseph Pilates. It refers to the center of the body which creates the foundation for all movement.

I trained intensively and my 'inner athlete' was happy again. In 2008 I was hired at Arbutus Club, the most prestigious private club in Vancouver, to teach mat Pilates. Starting with four classes, my vision of building this space into a full studio became real in a matter of one year. I left Noam Gagnon in 2009 to focus on starting the studio and soon was working sixty hours a week. I needed to hire other teachers, and in 2010 one more instructor joined my studio.

In January of 2010, Dean had a near-death experience due to a snowmobile accident in Squamish and ended up at the hospital with a concussion (it was the sixth one in his life). After a few days, the doctors let him leave but that was a huge mistake. He never followed up his doctor's sessions and for the next six months, I did not know who I was living with. One day he was the man I was going to marry, the next - a stranger who accused me of having affairs with my clients. He even changed the locks many times. I cried for six months. Finally, in September 2010, I decided to end my life. Thankfully, there was Bev who became not only my mentor but also a very close friend. She took me to Peru, to discover shamanic healing work. By this time, Bev was living part-time in Peru. She was starting a crystal business organizing personal soul quest retreats with clients. The time spent there was truly transformational for me. She connected me with a very well-known shaman Puma. I discovered Watchuma[7] work but was not ready for Ayahuasca[8] with master Pandero Bev had told me that everything would be different when I returned to Vancouver. I could not believe how right she was. When I came back, Dean was waiting with a suitcase of mine. I thought, "Well, he is ready to make this relationship work", but instead, he dropped me at the holiday inn on Broadway Avenue. I was left alone with no phone, no computer, no money, but I found peace in this heartbroken chaos. Two days later, I had to return to the Arbutus Club to teach, yet

---

[7] A plant cactus medicine with origins in ancient Andean Mountains of Peru used for prophecies and expansions of consciousness.

[8] Psychoactive brew used as a traditional spiritual medicine in ceremonies among the indigenous peoples of the Amazon basin.

I did not say a word. I started searching on Craigslist for rentals but became overwhelmed with looking at dumps, basements, and places where no cats were allowed. It was very important for me since, at that time, I was the owner of two Maine Coon cats. After a week of this nonsense, I put what I had learned from the shamans into practice and visualized where I wanted to live. The next morning I found the perfect place. I called the landlord and told him its mine without looking at it. He was stunned when I met him with a cheque in hand. I told him that I had two cats and that they are the love of my life. I also confessed that I needed a break, and due to my honesty, he accepted me.

In 2011 I returned to Peru and worked with master Pandero and Ayahuasca; I became a shaman and a certified teacher in shamanic Ashtanga[9] practice. I felt I finally was at peace and was attaining the physical, mental, and spiritual balance. I got rid of my issues and fears and started working on feeling love again. I was grateful for who I was, for the place where I was living, for teaching classical Pilates, and for the love of my life: Zia and Thor, feline siblings.

In September of the same year, I was devastated by the news of my ex-common-law relationship Robin committing suicide. It brought back memories and triggered my feelings and regrets that I have never managed to say in person. I was stronger by practicing shamanic work and Pilates. I realized that it was a god-given blessing that I had left him a few years ago as otherwise, I would have gone so far down that I probably would have never survived his death.

In 2013, I flew to Timbavati, and it was my first trip back to the country of Africa. I spent one month there, on the Global White Lion Protection Trust reserve[10]. I needed this powerful healing. Thanks to that divine journey, I was finally able to come to terms with my past and face up the fact of Robin's suicide.

---

[9] Ashtanga yoga is named after the term given in Patanjali's Yoga Sutras for the eight-fold path of yoga, or ashtanga, meaning "eight-limbed" in Sanskrit.

[10] A registered NPO/Public Benefit Organisation situated in a protected area of nearly 4,400 acres of endemic bushveld.

In the summer of 2014, after helping a client of mine, I suffered lower back pain and devastating side effects would imply. I was sure there was more in the classical Pilates work than Romana Kryzanowska trained so on July 1, 2014, I looked on the internet for the remaining elders that worked with Joe and I found Jay Grimes. I knew I had found my real purpose. However, I was wondering what I should do to work with him. Luckily, my friend Bev was close and she suggested I simply call LA. As I did it, my whole life changed.

I flew to LA the following week to see how I would train to pass the reformer assessment for 'The Work'[11] in 2015. After 10 days of intensive training, I was advised to wait until November, near the end date, to assess if I needed to train harder. I was crushed, but my 'inner athlete' was on fire.

At the same time, I took a three-month work permit to take a full-time classical teacher position at the only classical studio in Bermuda. On the spot, I found all the Gratz[12] equipment. Before I flew to Los Angeles, I had not been working on any Gratz equipment, and in my first private session, I did not have enough powerhouse to use it! Having the opportunity to train on these pieces allowed me to train better and pass my assessment.

2015 was the year of 'The Work' with Jay Grimes. During that period, my teaching, my understanding, and my practices changed completely. One of Jay's advice, right from the start of the mentorship program, was to give up running, biking, and swimming for one year to allow real changes in my body. I agreed without hesitation, knowing that it was the best decision I made. This was rare for a former professional athlete, but, deep down inside, I knew there was more to it. To allow deep changes in my body, I had to be patient, adaptable and committed to the journey ahead. I could not take

---

[11] An intensive one to two-year program for those who want to go beyond the workshop and truly understand how all the Pilates exercises and equipment work together efficiently and effectively.

[12] The original manufacturer of Pilates apparatus.

shortcuts as my body needed time to change from years of abusing it. I was a completely different person and teacher. After I completed 'The Work' in the winter of 2015, I went out and bought new running shoes as I wanted to test my condition. One block away, I stopped and asked myself, "What is wrong?". So I returned to the running store and bought shoes for walking instead. I finally listened to my body and disliked the chaotic feeling in it. I started practicing daily and taking private lessons several times a week. I was in heaven and my body was changing!

I became stronger again but with more inner deep muscles of the powerhouse while finding more balance with the flexibility and more control of my mind. I learned that the powerhouse is much more than just the stomach and that there is a two-way stretch in the back and at the front of the body. My posture changed from an upper rounded back to an even taller upper middle back where my tightness was accumulated from years of Ironman training and sports. Also, my quadricepses became more balanced with my hamstrings and I was having fewer tugs in hip flexors. I was feeling my buttocks working in a lengthening contraction instead of a squeezing. I allowed the whole body to work evenly instead of focusing on the extremities. I became more balanced in my ways of standing, walking, and sitting. My mild tear completely disappeared and healed from lengthening these muscles upwards instead of being pushed downwards. I felt a sense of childlike play, just like when I was back in Africa playing with my chimpanzee Catherine. My head was more on top of my torso instead of forwarding, hyperextending my neck even more. It became clearer that all the other fitness activities I was doing were not what my body needed anymore. I quit everything to do just classical work from Joe's teachings. I saw things differently. I even had a stronger bond connection with my two Maine Coon cats. I became more grounded and peaceful. I made the right choices and was looking at life on a deeper level.

In 2016 in Whistler, during a weekend workshop with Karen Frishmann, I met a new polish teacher, Mariola, who invited me to Poland. The same year I re-branded my business with the help of Bev, who came up with the name "Lineage Pilates". I also made the bold decision to quit the prestigious private club to be on my own.

Mariola fell in love with classical Pilates and my teaching. In 2017 I flew to Warsaw for the weekend conference where I met 25 teachers, all craving this work. Mariola took me to Kraków and Lublin, her hometown, where we talked about finally opening the first classical studio in Poland.

In 2018 I started Lineage Pilates comprehensive teacher training lasting eighteen months and flew five times to Lublin, Poland, where "Klasyczny Pilates" studio with two groups of teachers was born.

That year I changed teacher and started training with Samantha Walley who was the first teacher to enter the work with Jay Grimes in 2011. She completely changed the way I was looking at the work by going deeper into it. She made me a better teacher and gave what I was looking for which was depth in training and not just move and exercise. I knew this system so well but still, I had a missing link of connecting the body to the mind. Samantha had been a scientist by trade before she became a master Pilates teacher and I was searching for the science part of it. My body changed even more with peeling off the deep layers of the upper and middle back realigning my rib cage, lengthening my low back, and finding new strength in my upper back connection. She allowed me to feel the pathways of the muscles going down and up. As Jay Grimes would say, "Think with your body and feel with your mind". I finally learned through movement. Once my body was aligned, it opened muscle pathways, which later lifted to the neck, head, and brain. It allowed the body to feel the missing link connection of the powerhouse. The body works as ONE enabling emotion to surface and then to release. In being able to truly find closure with emotions, it needs to pass through you and you should feel it before letting it go. I was also able to go through peri and menopause with ease. I accepted my body changing and aging but by getting stronger, leaner, and with almost no aches and pains. I still have big goals that I want to achieve, no matter the age.

In March of 2018, I was involved in a near-death car accident from not wearing my back seat belt and went flying into the passenger door. I ended up suffering from pulled ribs, a crooked neck, and a shoulder injury. For nine months, I was not able to do a push-up or practice the advanced work of the Pilates system. Instead, I believed in this technique, and it made me search for the mind component into the body relationship. Without Samantha's guidance in bringing more depth to this system, I would have still been struggling with this huge setback. I think that injuries, setbacks, or accidents are the best lessons as they made me who I am today as a teacher and person. I believe in the impossible and with commitment, dedication, resilience, and trust everything is possible. The mind is so powerful.

In 2019, after the death of Zia - my second Maine Coon - I decided to pack up and start a new life in Poland. The year before, when Thor passed away, I decided to move all my equipment into my apartment as Zia was now alone. For eighteen years, she and her brother were inseparable so I did not want to waste more time teaching away from home for too long and instead had my clients come to me. I became homebound and spent every evening with her. My clients all loved her and the feline energy was part of the Pilates practice in everyone. In the fall of 2019, she stopped eating, and, after a visit to my holistic vet, she had only weeks to live. I was devastated but so happy that I was able to stay with her twenty-four hours a day. I did not want to let her go but the time came where I had to make the call. I felt her last heartbeat and with Thor - his last breath. Both, to this day, are still in my heart. After Zia's death, I was left alone for the first time in my entire life without a man or an animal. I got used to being single but I was not sure if I could be without my Maine Coons. It was a very testing time for me. I was struggling with myself not to go back into the abyss of wanting to take my life as I had nothing to look forward to. I was left only with Pilates and I have to admit that it saved my life. I believe that I have never found true love with a man, but I did found it with Thor and Zia, and that is enough.

I moved from Lublin to Warsaw in the middle of 2019 to train the third group of teachers through "Sense Studio", a private club run by the top ten millionaire businessman in Poland. I was featured in *Vogue* and gave several interviews spreading the Joseph Pilates method all over Poland and the world.

When the Covid epidemic came in March of 2020, I became adaptable. Instead of fighting these hard times, I brought my Lineage Pilates fully online and set up my private Facebook page "Total Body Transformation For Women Over 40: Lineage Pilates" as well as my first online program "The Essential Powerhouse" and about to launch my second online program called "Classical Pilates Quest" six weeks program. I started my Ladysmith group of ladies that joined me when I was a brand new teacher back in 2004 when I opened my first studio. As a teacher, you meet many people who become your clients for life, and these ladies have been a huge part of my path, always reconnecting when a breakthrough happens. That is a very special bond since they all needed the method of Pilates to lift their spirits and to find the zest for life through moving on the mat. They taught me to truly challenge my knowledge by finding the 'equipment from the studio' in house furniture and teaching this system with what they have. These times truly showed my growth as a teacher and my compassion for what Joe created while he was on the island of men during World War One. He was kept there in jail, with cold walls and inmates dying of malnutrition. Thus, he started the mat routine known as classical Pilates and after his release four years later, he created the Reformer, an apparatus with springs to help find the spring in your center. The rest of the equipment came soon after.

I practice six days a week, keeping my zest for life, and I teach fully online. I know that I was meant to be alive and it becomes clearer during Covid times that this method is a must to practice for everyone. It saved my life physically, mentally, emotionally, and spiritually.

www.lineagepilates.com
Total Body Transformation For Women Over 40: Lineage Pilates

https://www.facebook.com/groups/2716553805222905/

Email
Jacqueline@lineagepilates.com

Facebook
Jacqueline Martin
https://www.facebook.com/jacqueline.martin.798278

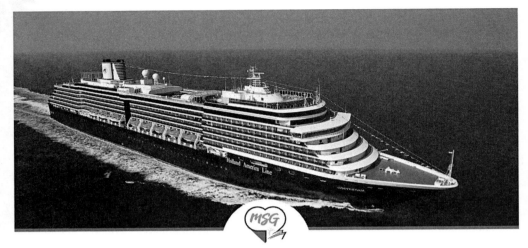

HARRIS HOLIDAY CRUISES

Harris Holiday Cruises Celebrating Life's Transitional Seasons

At HARRIS HOLIDAY CRUISES, our cruises offer worthwhile travelling experiences that inspire, educate, encourage, and build strong relationships among our global sisterhood. We are a community of accomplished women eager to have fun while marking a significant milestone. Our vision is to globally change the imprint for women feeling invisible through education, inspiration and a loving supportive community. Our special interest cruises will carry forth this vision with the support of our council of experts who have joined our team.

HTTPS://WWW.HARRISHOLIDAYCRUISES.COM/

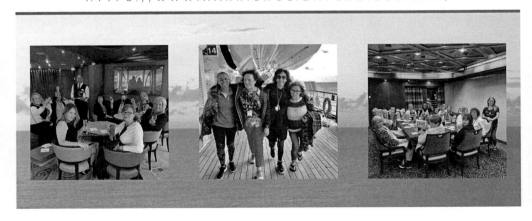